CRQs in Anaesthesia

Constructed Response Questions for Exams

Thanthullu Vasu
Mahesh Kodivalasa
Pradeep Mukund Ingle
Mehar Ahson
Lohita Rilesh Nanda

tfm Publishing Limited, Castle Hill Barns, Harley, Shrewsbury, SY5 6LX, UK
Tel: +44 (0)1952 510061; Fax: +44 (0)1952 510192
E-mail: info@tfmpublishing.com; Web site: www.tfmpublishing.com

Editing, design & typesetting: Nikki Bramhill BSc Hons Dip Law
Cover photo: © iStock.com
Anesthesia machine in hospital operating room
Credit: lyosha_nazarenko; stock photo ID: 627431634

First edition:	© 2019
Paperback	ISBN: 978-1-910079-79-9
E-book editions:	© 2019
ePub	ISBN: 978-1-910079-80-5
Mobi	ISBN: 978-1-910079-81-2
Web pdf	ISBN: 978-1-910079-82-9

Printed by Gutenberg Press Ltd., Gudja Road, Tarxien, GXQ 2902, Malta
Tel: +356 2398 2201; Fax: +356 2398 2290
E-mail: info@gutenberg.com.mt; Web site: www.gutenberg.com.mt

Contents

Chapter 5 Cardiac anaesthesia QUESTIONS

Chapter 6 Intensive care QUESTIONS

Chapter 7 Perioperative medicine QUESTIONS

Chapter 8 Regional, orthopaedic and trauma anaesthesia QUESTIONS

Chapter 9 Other topics in general medicine QUESTIONS

Chapter 13 Paediatric anaesthesia ANSWERS

Chapter 14 Pain ANSWERS

Chapter 15 Cardiac anaesthesia ANSWERS

Chapter 16 Intensive care ANSWERS

Chapter 17 Perioperative medicine ANSWERS

Chapter 18 Regional, orthopaedic and trauma anaesthesia ANSWERS

Chapter 19 Other topics in general medicine ANSWERS

Preface

Examinations are a stressful experience for many, but it is a recognised way of assessing our knowledge. The final FRCA exams from the Royal College of Anaesthetists have an international reputation and the College is committed to maintaining the highest possible standards for its exams. Recently, based on the 2015 exam review (as approved by the General Medical Council), the College introduced constructed response questions (CRQs) to replace the short answer questions. The reason for this change was that the College wanted to assess not only a candidate's knowledge and understanding, but also the *application* of the knowledge and possibly evaluation and judgement. CRQs help to achieve this goal.

CRQs have more subsections and are specific in their required responses. The examiners can get an exact indication of what answers to accept or not. Candidates are required to read the questions and answer closely with regard to what has been specifically asked.

"We are what we repeatedly do.
Excellence, then, is not an act, but a habit."
Aristotle

Practising with past papers is vital in any exam preparation. CRQs will be introduced to the exams from September 2019 and we are proud that this is one of the first books to be produced for this purpose. We have tried to simulate the Royal College papers and have extensively researched recent *BJA Education* papers, e-learning, CEPD resources and other vital educational materials to select the appropriate topics.

This book tests with a similar pattern to that of the Royal College exams. One hundred and thirty-four questions have been produced in a similar ratio to the subsections in exams. In the FRCA exam, there will be a total of 12 questions, one each from the six mandatory units of training (neuroanaesthesia; obstetric anaesthesia; paediatric anaesthesia; pain; cardiac anaesthesia; and intensive care), and six from general duties which may include one from optional unit training (perioperative medicine; regional, orthopaedic and trauma anaesthesia; other topics in general medicine; and optional topics). If you have practised this entire book, you should have at least covered 11 FRCA question papers! To make it easy for the revising candidate, we have split the questions into their respective subspecialty topics, so the reader can assess their knowledge appropriately in a timely manner. The answers are only an example and we advise candidates to use the references and resources for further update.

The Royal College of Anaesthetists conducted CRQ pilot exams in January and June 2018; unfortunately, the pass rate (44.33%) was less than that expected from the similar short answer format (50-60%). The reasons assumed included: a failure to answer the question that was specifically asked, a poor knowledge of pathophysiology, a failure to prioritise answers, etc. If a question asks for any four causes, there will only be four blanks to fill the answers and candidates need to remember what to prioritise. Further, the pass rate was much less in pain, intensive care and obstetric topics. We strongly advise candidates to practise the questions in an exam-simulated environment and then reassess themselves with the model answers provided in the second half of the book.

I thank all my co-authors Mahesh, Pradeep, Lohita and Mehar who have worked hard to make sure that this book is a successful and useful aid to all anaesthetists.

We thank you for purchasing this book and wish you all the best in your forthcoming exams and endeavours.

Dr. Thanthullu Vasu
Consultant and Lead for Intermediate teaching
University Hospitals of Leicester NHS Trust
vasubangor@gmail.com

Foreword

Anaesthesia training in the UK has undergone many organisational and politically driven changes. The anaesthesia specialty has maintained its academic and professional standards and has emerged to be one of the disciplines that offers the safest clinical care. A career in anaesthesia is not for the faint-hearted. Apart from achieving competency in different areas of training, trainees have to be successful in the demanding exams. The Royal College exams can be challenging because of the enormity of the curriculum and the high standards expected.

Constructed response questions (CRQs) are a relatively newer way of assessment. CRQs are used for higher-order thinking skills such as analysis and evaluation. Commonly, these questions provide trainees with a prompt and require them to write a structured answer. The ability to extract information from the prompt forms the basis for answering the question. The Royal College of Anaesthetists is in the process of moving away from short answer questions to CRQs. The objective is to assess not only the knowledge and understanding but also the application of knowledge and possibly evaluation and judgement.

Dr. Vasu and his team have excellent academic and teaching credentials. They have been successfully running different exam preparation courses and have used their vast experience and resources to prepare this book on CRQs. In line with the examination syllabus, the book contains six core modules (neuroanaesthesia, obstetrics, paediatrics, cardiac anaesthesia, pain and intensive care), general modules and optional unit questions. The second part of the book provides model answers to the questions in each module.

tfm publishing has a rich experience in publishing high-quality medical books and has a track record of producing many successful exam preparation materials. This book on CRQs will be a valuable contribution and useful guide for anaesthesia trainees preparing for the highly competitive exam as well as experienced trainers actively involved in teaching.

Dr. Shyam Balasubramanian
Consultant in Pain Medicine and Anaesthesia
University Hospitals of Coventry and Warwickshire
Regional Adviser for Pain Medicine, West Midlands
Editor *BJA Education* (2011-16)
Member, Professional Standards Committee, Faculty of Pain Medicine

Contributors

Dr. Thanthullu Vasu MBBS MD DNB FRCA FFPMRCA Dip Pain Mgt
Consultant in Pain Medicine, University Hospitals of Leicester NHS Trust, UK

Dr. Mahesh Kodivalasa MBBS MD FRCA FFPMRCA
Consultant in Anaesthetics and Pain Medicine, University Hospitals of Leicester NHS Trust, UK

Dr. Pradeep Mukund Ingle MBBS MD Dip Critical Care FRCA FFPMRCA
Consultant in Anaesthetics and Pain Medicine, University Hospitals of North Midlands, Stoke-on-Trent, UK

Dr. Mehar Ahson MBBS MD FRCA
ST7 trainee in Anaesthetics, East Midlands School of Anaesthesia, UK

Dr. Lohita Rilesh Nanda MBBS MD FRCA
ST7 trainee in Anaesthetics, East Midlands School of Anaesthesia, UK

Acknowledgements

Thanks to Nikki Bramhill, tfm publishing Ltd, for her constant support and encouragement in making this book possible. tfm publishing Ltd has supported us from the initial idea right through to making this a reality. No words are enough to thank Nikki for her professionalism and skills.

We thank Dr. Ravindra Pochiraju MBBS MD EDIC FFICM, Leicester Royal Infirmary, for preparing the intensive care questions 1 to 5.

Abbreviations

5-HT	5-hydroxytryptamine or serotonin
AAA	Abdominal aortic aneurysm
AAG	Alpha-1 acid glycoprotein
AAGA	Accidental awareness under general anaesthesia
AAGBI	Association of Anaesthetists of Great Britain and Ireland
ABC	Airway, breathing, circulation approach
ABCDE	Airway, breathing, circulation, disability and exposure
ABG	Arterial blood gas
AC	Alternating current
ACE	Angiotensin converting enzyme
ACR	Acute cellular rejection
ACS	Acute coronary syndrome
ACS NSQIP	American College of Surgeons National Surgical Quality Improvement Program
ACT	Activated coagulation time
ACTH	Adrenocorticotropic hormone
ADH	Antidiuretic hormone
ADL	Activities of daily living
ADP	Adenosine diphosphate
AED	Antiepileptic drug
AF	Atrial fibrillaton
AFE	Amniotic fluid embolism
AFOI	Awake fibreoptic intubation
AKI	Acute kidney injury
ALI	Acute lung injury
ALS®	Advanced Life Support
AMR	Antibody-mediated rejection
APACHE	Acute Physiology and Chronic Health Evaluation
APH	Antepartum haemorrhage

APL	Adjustable pressure-limiting
Ar^+	Argon
ARDS	Acute respiratory distress syndrome
ARIS-CAT	Assess Respiratory risk In Surgical patients in CATalonia (score)
ASA	American Society of Anesthesiologists
ASA-PS	American Society of Anesthesiologists Physical Status (score)
ASD	Atrial septal defect
ASRA	American Society of Regional Anesthesia
AT	Anaerobic threshold
ATLS®	Advanced Trauma Life Support
ATP	Adenosine triphosphate
AVPU	Alert, Verbal, Pain, Unresponsive (scale)
AVR	Aortic valve replacement
BCIS	Bone cement implantation syndrome
BD	*bis in die*; twice daily
BiPAP	Biphasic positive airway pressure
BIS	Bispectral index (monitoring)
BMI	Body Mass Index
BP	Blood pressure
BPI	Brief Pain Inventory
CABG	Coronary artery bypass graft
CAM-ICU	Confusion Assessment Method for the Intensive Care Unit
cAMP	Cyclic adenosine monophosphate
CBG	Capillary blood glucose
CCF	Congestive cardiac failure
cGMP	Cyclic guanosine monophosphate
CICV	Can't intubate and can't ventilate
CK	Creatine kinase
CMP	Case Mix Programme
CMV	*Cytomegalovirus*
CNS	Central nervous system
CO_2	Carbon dioxide
COPD	Chronic obstructive pulmonary disease
COX	Cyclo-oxygenase

CP	Cerebral palsy
CPAP	Continuous positive airway pressure
CPB	Cardiopulmonary bypass
CPET	Cardiopulmonary exercise testing
CPP	Cerebral perfusion pressure
CPR	Cardiopulmonary resuscitation
CRF	Chronic renal failure
CRP	C-reactive protein
CRPS	Complex regional pain syndrome
CRRT	Continuous renal replacement therapy
CSE	Combined spinal-epidural
CSF	Cerebrospinal fluid
CT	Computed tomography
CTG	Cardiotocography
CTZ	Chemoreceptor trigger zone
CVA	Cerebrovascular accident
CVP	Central venous pressure
CVS	Cardiovascular system
CVVH	Continuous veno-venous haemofiltration
CVVHD	Continuous veno-venous haemodialysis
CVVHDF	Continuous veno-venous haemodiafiltration
CXR	Chest X-ray
CYP	Cytochrome peroxidase enzyme
DAS	Difficult Airway Society
DCM	Dilated cardiomyopathy
DHPR	Dihydropyridine receptor
DI	Diabetes insipidus
DIC	Disseminated intravascular coagulation
DIEP	Deep inferior epigastric perforator
DKA	Diabetic ketoacidosis
DLCO	Diffusing capacity of lung for carbon monoxide
DLT	Double-lumen tube
DM	Diabetes mellitus
DMARD	Disease-modifying antirheumatic drug

DN4	Douleur Neuropathique 4
DNA	Deoxyribonucleic acid
DOAC	Direct oral anticoagulant
DPP-4	Dipeptidyl peptidase-4
DRWR	Donor-recipient weight ratio
DSM	Diagnostic and Statistical Manual of Mental Disorders
DVT	Deep venous thrombosis
EBGD	Evidence-based guideline development
EBP	Epidural blood patch
EBV	Ebstein-Barr virus
EC	Excitation-contraction
ECG	Electrocardiograph
ECMO	Extracorporeal membrane oxygenation
EEG	Electroencephalograph
eGFR	Estimated glomerular filtration rate
ELPQuiC	Emergency Laparotomy Pathway Quality Improvement Care
EMG	Electromyography
EMLA	Eutectic mixture of local anaesthetics
ENT	Ear, nose and throat
E-PASS	Estimation of Physiological Ability and Surgical Stress
ERAS	Enhanced recovery after surgery
ERCP	Endoscopic retrograde cholangiopancreatogram
ERP	Enhanced recovery programme
ESRF	End-stage renal failure
$etCO_2$	End-tidal carbon dioxide
ETT	Endotracheal tube
EVAR	Endovascular aneurysm repair
FBC	Full blood count
FEV1	Forced expiratory volume in 1 second
FHR	Foetal heart rate
FiO_2	Fraction of inspired oxygen
FLACC	Face, Legs, Activity, Cry, Consolability (scale)
FRC	Functional residual capacity
FVC	Forced vital capacity
GA	General anaesthesia

GaAs	Gallium arsenide
GABA	Gamma aminobutyric acid
GBS	Guillain-Barré syndrome
GCS	Glasgow Coma Scale
GDT	Goal-directed therapy
GFR	Glomerular filtration rate
GH	Growth hormone
GI	Gastrointestinal
GLP-1	Glucagon-like peptide-1
GMC	General Medical Council
GOLD	Global initiative for chronic Obstructive Lung Disease
GORD	Gastro-oesophageal reflux disease
GP	Glycoprotein
GTN	Glyceryl trinitrate
H/o	History of
Hb	Haemoglobin
HDU	High dependency unit
HELLP	Haemolysis (H); elevated liver enzymes (EL); low platelets (LP)
HFOV	High-frequency oscillation ventilation
Hg	Mercury
Hib	*Haemophilus influenzae* type b
HIV	Human immunodeficiency virus
HLA	Human leucocyte antigen
HPA axis	Hypothalamopituitary adrenal axis
HR	Heart rate
HRA	Health and Research Authority
HSV	*Herpes simplex* virus
HTN	Hypertension
HZV	*Herpes zoster* virus
IAH	Intra-abdominal hypertension
IBW	Ideal body weight
ICD	Implantable cardioverter defibrillator
ICDSC	Intensive Care Delirium Screening Checklist
ICNARC	Intensive Care National Audit and Research Centre
ICP	Intracranial pressure

ICS	Intensive Care Society
ICU	Intensive care unit
IgE	Immunoglobulin E
IHD	Ischaemic heart disease
ILE	Intravenous lipid emulsion
IM	Intramuscular
INR	International Normalised Ratio
IPH	Inadvertent perioperative hypothermia
IPPV	Intermittent positive pressure ventilation
ISHLT	International Registry of Paediatric Heart and Lung Transplantation
IT	Intrathecal
ITDD	Intrathecal drug delivery
ITU	Intensive therapy unit
IUFD	Intrauterine foetal death
IUGR	Intrauterine growth retardation
IV	Intravenous
IVC	Inferior vena cava
kPa	Kilopascal
KTP	Potassium titanyl phosphate laser
LA	Local anaesthesia
LANSS	Leeds Assessment of Neuropathic Symptoms and Signs Scale
LASER	Light amplification by stimulated emission of radiation
LAST	Local anaesthetic systemic toxicity
LD	Latissimus dorsi
LDH	Lactate dehydrogenase
LFT	Liver function test
LLN	Lower limit of normal
LMA	Laryngeal mask airway
LMWH	Low-molecular-weight heparin
LOS	Lower oesophageal sphincter
LSCS	Lower segment caesarean section
LV	Left ventricle
LVH	Left ventricular hypertrophy
LVRS	Lung volume reduction surgery

MAP	Mean arterial pressure
MBRRACE	Mothers and Babies: Reducing Risk through Audits and Confidential Enquiries
MCA	Mental Capacity Act
MDT	Multidisciplinary team
MEOWS	Modified Early Obstetric Warning Score
MEP	Motor evoked potential
mg	Milligram
MH	Malignant hyperthermia
MI	Myocardial infarction
MIBG	Metaiodo-benzylguanidine (scan)
MRC	Medical Research Council
MRI	Magnetic resonance imaging
MS	Mitral stenosis
MVV	Maximal voluntary ventilation
NAP	National Audit Project
NCEPOD	National Confidential Enquiry into Patient Outcome and Death
NCS	Nerve conduction study
NDMR	Non-depolarising muscle relaxant
Nd-YAG	Neodymium yttrium aluminium oxide garnet laser
NELA	National Emergency Laparotomy Audit
NEWS	National Early Warning Score
NG	Nasogastric
NHS	National Health Service
NIBP	Non-invasive blood pressure
NICE	National Institute for Health and Care Excellence
NICU	Neonatal intensive care unit
NIRS	Near infrared spectroscopy
NMBA	Neuromuscular blocking agent
NMDA	N-methyl-D-aspartate
NNH	Numbers needed to harm
NNT	Numbers needed to treat
NO	Nitric oxide

NPSA	National Patient Safety Agency
NRS	Numerical Rating Scale
NSAID	Non-steroidal anti-inflammatory drug
O_2	Oxygen
OGD	Oesophagogastroduodenoscopy
OIH	Opioid-induced hyperalgesia
OLV	One-lung ventilation
OPCAB	Off-pump coronary artery bypass
OSA	Obstructive sleep apnoea
OxyHb	Oxyhaemoglobin
P/F	PaO_2/FiO_2
p50	Partial pressure at 50% saturation
PA catheter	Pulmonary artery catheter
$PACO_2$	Alveolar partial pressure of carbon dioxide
$PaCO_2$	Arterial partial pressure of carbon dioxide
PaO_2	Partial pressure of arterial oxygen
PAR	Protease activated receptor
PCA	Patient-controlled analgesia
PCEA	Patient-controlled epidural analgesia
PCI	Percutaneous coronary intervention
pCO_2	Partial pressure of carbon dioxide
PCR	Polymerase chain reaction
PDE	Phosphodiesterase
PDPH	Postdural puncture headache
PE	Pulmonary embolism
PECS	Pectoralis block
PEEP	Positive end-expiratory pressure
PEG	Percutaneous endoscopic gastrostomy
PET	Positive emission tomography
PFTs	Pulmonary function tests
pH	Measurement of logarithmic concentration of hydrogen ions
PICC	Peripherally inserted central catheters
PICU	Paediatric intensive care unit
PIH	Pregnancy-induced hypertension

PiO_2	Inspired partial pressure of oxygen
pO_2	Partial pressure of oxygen
PONV	Postoperative nausea and vomiting
POSSUM	Physiological and Operative Severity Score for the enUmeration of Mortality and morbidity
PPH	Postpartum haemorrhage
PPM	Permanent pacemaker
ppo	Predicted postoperative
P-POSSUM	Portsmouth POSSUM
PR	Per rectum
PRA	Panel reactive antibody
PRIS	Propofol-related infusion syndrome
PRN	*Pro re nata* (when necessary or as and when needed)
PT	Prothrombin time
PTLD	Post-transplant lymphoproliferative disease
PVR	Pulmonary vascular resistance
QDS	*quater die sumendum*; four times a day
qSOFA	Quick Sequential Organ Failure Assessment
RA	Regional anaesthesia
RCoA	Royal College of Anaesthetists
RCRI	Revised Cardiac Risk Index
RCT	Randomised controlled trial
RF	Radiofrequency
RhA	Rheumatoid arthritis
ROTEM®	Rotational thromboelastometry
RQ	Respiratory quotient
RR	Respiratory rate
RRT	Renal replacement therapy
RSI	Rapid sequence induction
RV	Right ventricle
RyR	Ryanodine receptor isoform
SAD	Supraglottic airway device
SAH	Subarachnoid haemorrhage
SALT	Speech and language therapy

SCS	Spinal cord stimulator
SCUF	Slow continuous ultrafiltration
SIADH	Syndrome of inappropriate antidiuretic hormone
SICSQIG	Scottish Intensive Care Society Quality Improvement Group
SIGN	Scottish Intercollegiate Guidelines Network
SIRS	Systemic inflammatory response syndrome
SLE	Systemic lupus erythematosus
SMR	Standardised mortality ratio
SNP	Sodium nitroprusside
SNRI	Serotonin norepinephrine reuptake inhibitor
SOFA	Sequential Organ Failure Assessment
SORT	Surgical Outcome Risk Tool
SpO_2	Peripheral capillary oxygen saturation
SRS	Surgical Risk Scale
SSEP	Somatosensory evoked potential
SSI	Surgical site infection
SVR	Systemic vascular resistance
SVT	Supraventricular tachycardia
TACO	Transfusion-associated circulatory overload
TAP	Transverse abdominis plane (block)
TBI	Traumatic brain injury
TCI	Target-controlled infusion
TDS	*ter die sumendum*; three times a day
TED™	Thromboembolism deterrent (stockings)
TEG®	Thromboelastography
TENS	Transcutaneous electrical nerve stimulation
TIA	Transient ischaemic attack
TIVA	Total intravenous anaesthesia
TLCO	Transfer factor for lung carbon monoxide (synonymous with DLCO)
TMJ	Temporomandibular joint
TNF	Tumour necrosis factor
TOE	Transoesophageal echocardiogram
TOF	Tetrology of Fallot

TORCH	Toxoplasmosis, Rubella, Cytomegalovirus, Herpes virus infections
TPN	Total parenteral nutrition
TRALI	Transfusion-related lung injury
TRAM	Transverse rectus abdominis myocutaneous flap
TRIM	Transfusion-related (associated) immunomodulation
TRPV	Transient receptor potential (cation) vanilloid
TSH	Thyroid-stimulating hormone
TT	Thrombin time
TTE	Transthoracic echocardiogram
US	Ultrasound
UKOSS	UK Obstetric Surveillance System
V/Q ratio	Ventilation/Perfusion ratio
V/Q scan	Ventilation/Perfusion scan
VAP	Ventilator-associated pneumonia
VAS	Visual Analogue Scale
VATS	Video-assisted thoracoscopic surgery
VBA	Very Brief Advice (tool)
VE	Ventilatory equivalent
VF	Ventricular fibrillation
VR	Ventilatory reserve
VRS	Verbal Rating Scale
VSD	Ventricular septal defect
VT	Ventricular tachycardia
VTE	Venous thromboembolism
vWF	von-Willebrand factor
WBC	White blood cell
WHO	World Health Organisation

Section 1
Questions

Chapter 1

Neuroanaesthesia

QUESTIONS

Q1 — Cerebrospinal fluid physiology

a) Describe the production and circulation of cerebrospinal fluid (CSF). 3 marks

b) How does the intracranial pressure affect the production and absorption of CSF? 2 marks

c) Give five differentiating features of CSF vs. plasma with regards to its biochemistry. 5 marks

d) List any four indications for lumbar puncture. 4 marks

e) Name any six factors that predispose to the development of a postdural puncture headache after lumbar puncture. 6 marks

Q2 — Brainstem death and organ donation

A 20-year-old patient in a neurointensive care unit satisfies the criteria for brainstem death and has been accepted as an organ donor.

a) List the main adverse cardiovascular changes associated with brainstem death. 5 marks

b) What are the physiological goals (with values) required to ensure optimisation of this donor? 7 marks

c) Outline the measures that may be used to achieve the needed goals. 5 marks

d) Name any three medications that you might use to optimise the endocrine system. 3 marks

Q3 — Status epilepticus

You are asked to review a 27-year-old male who is a known epileptic in convulsive status epilepticus.

a) Name two opioids contraindicated in seizures. 2 marks

b) What are the implications of neuromuscular blocking drugs in epileptic patients? 2 marks

c) Define convulsive status epilepticus. 1 mark

d) What drugs, including doses, are used during the various stages of status epilepticus? 5 marks

Premonitory stage: ______________________________
(prehospital or <5 minutes)

Early stage: ______________________________
(5-10 minutes)

Established stage: ______________________________
(0-60 minutes)

e) What investigations would you consider in a patient with status epilepticus? 2 marks

f) Sixty minutes after your initial management, the patient continues to be in status epilepticus. What would be your further management? 5 marks

g) What are the complications associated with refractory convulsive status epilepticus? 3 marks

Q4 — Delirium in critical care

a) Define delirium. 2 marks

b) List the key clinical features that are used to diagnose delirium in critical care. 4 marks

c) List any six risk factors for delirium in an intensive care patient. 3 marks

d) List some methods of diagnosis and assessment of delirium. 1 mark

e) In a delirious critical care patient, what are the most common environmental factors that are potentially treatable? 3 marks

f) What medical factors would you correct to treat/prevent delirium? 3 marks

g) When is pharmacological treatment indicated and which classes of drugs can be used? 4 marks

Q5 — Near-drowning

A 20-year-old man is brought to the emergency department having been pulled from a river following a near-drowning.

a) What are the effects of near-drowning on the respiratory and cardiovascular systems? 2 marks

b) What are the effects on other systems? 1 mark

c) List the relevant features in the history that you would elicit in this patient. 3 marks

d) List the investigations that you would perform in this particular patient. 3 marks

e) How would you treat hypothermia in this patient? 4 marks

f) What are the considerations for ventilatory strategies for this patient? 4 marks

g) Outline your neuroprotective strategies for this patient. 3 marks

Q6 — Acromegaly and hypophysectomy

A 54-year-old male with acromegaly presents for a transsphenoidal hypophysectomy.

a) What is acromegaly? 1 mark

b) List the clinical features of acromegaly which are of relevance to the anaesthetist. 3 marks

Airway: ____

Respiratory system: ______________________________________

Cardiovascular system: ___________________________________

c) What are the endocrine manifestations of pituitary adenomas? 1 mark

d) What other clinical presentations of a pituitary adenoma may be encountered? 2 marks

e) What are the specific preoperative considerations for anaesthetising this patient? 4 marks

f) What are your considerations during induction of anaesthesia for this patient? 2 marks

g) What are your concerns during maintenance of anaesthesia and emergence? 3 marks

h) What are the postoperative considerations after a transsphenoidal hypophysectomy? 2 marks

i) What are the advantages and disadvantages of a transsphenoidal hypophysectomy approach? 2 marks

Q7 — Intracranial pressure physiology

a) What is a normal intracranial pressure (ICP)? 2 marks

b) Describe a normal ICP waveform. 3 marks

c) How does the waveform change with increased ICP? 3 marks

d) What are the anatomical compensatory changes to a raised ICP? 4 marks

e) What are the symptoms and signs of a raised ICP? 4 marks

f) List the methods to monitor ICP in the intensive care unit. 4 marks

Q8 — Cerebral oxygenation and metabolism

A 59-year-old male is admitted in the neurocritical care unit with a head injury. He has an intraventricular bolt inserted for monitoring and measurement of intracranial pressure.

a) What are the advantages and disadvantages of measuring ICP using an intraventricular catheter? 4 marks

b) How is cerberal perfusion pressure (CPP) calculated? What is the optimal value recommended for favourable outcomes in intensive care? At what level must the transducers be zeroed to measure CPP? 3 marks

c) What are the methods used to measure cerebral oxygenation? What are the principles and the clinical applications? 3 marks

d) What are the methods used to measure cerebral blood flow? 3 marks

e) What are the clinical applications of transcranial Doppler? 3 marks

f) How is cerebral metabolism monitored? What are the substrates measured? 4 marks

Q9 — Posterior fossa tumour and air embolism

A 34-year-old man is scheduled for a posterior fossa tumour excision.

a) List four patient positions that might be employed for this operation. 2 marks

b) List five potential intraoperative and two postoperative problems that are associated with a posterior fossa craniotomy. 4 marks

c) What is the mechanism of cardiovascular instability in posterior cranial fossa tumour surgery? 2 marks

d) What are the contraindications to the sitting position? 2 marks

e) What monitoring techniques can specifically detect the presence of venous air embolism during surgery? For each method used, give the features that would indicate the diagnosis. 6 marks

f) How would you manage a significant venous air embolism in this patient? 4 marks

Q10 — Neuroradiology anaesthesia

An adult patient requires angiography and interventional radiology for a cerebral aneurysm.

a) List any six intracranial neuroradiological procedures. 3 marks

b) What potential problems may be encountered while anaesthetising a patient in the angiography suite? 3 marks

c) What are the specific preoperative anaesthetic considerations? 3 marks

d) What are the intraoperative anaesthetic considerations? 3 marks

e) Outline your management if haemorrhage occurs during the procedure. 3 marks

f) What are the effects of a subarachnoid haemorrhage on the cardiovascular and respiratory systems? What are the metabolic derangements? 5 marks

Chapter 2

Obstetric anaesthesia

QUESTIONS

Q1 — Pre-eclampsia

A 25-year-old woman who is 37 weeks pregnant and known to have pre-eclampsia is admitted to the labour ward with a blood pressure of 160/110mmHg on several readings.

a) What is the definition of pre-eclampsia? 1 mark

b) Define gestational hypertension. 1 mark

c) How can you define severe pre-eclampsia? 2 marks

d) Explain the pathogenesis of pre-eclampsia. 2 marks

e) Which related symptoms should pregnant women be told to report immediately? 2 marks

f) How should this patient be monitored following admission to the labour ward? 2 marks

g) How would you control BP in this patient? 2 marks

h) What changes would you make to your airway management for a pregnant woman, if this woman needed a general anaesthetic for a caesarean section? 3 marks

i) What are the other considerations for GA? 3 marks

j) What are the complications of pre-eclampsia? 2 marks

Q2 — Postdural puncture headache

The obstetric team tell you about a patient who is 2 days postpartum with a suspicion of a postdural puncture headache (PDPH).

a) What is the differential diagnosis for this patient with a suspected postpartum headache? 3 marks

b) What features, in this patient, would lead you to consider a serious underlying cause? 3 marks

c) What is the mechanism/pathogenesis of headache in PDPH? 1 mark

d) List the clinical features of PDPH. 2 marks

e) List the management strategies for this patient who is suffering with a PDPH. 4 marks

f) You diagnose a PDPH and arrange treatment by an epidural blood patch (EBP). How is an epidural blood patch performed? 2 marks

g) What advice would you give to the patient after an EBP? 1 mark

h) Describe the mechanism of action of an EBP. 1 mark

i) What are the described risks of an EBP? 3 marks

Q3 — Spinal anaesthesia for a caesarean section

a) Which methods of testing may be used to confirm the adequacy of a spinal (intrathecal) block for an elective caesarean section? 6 marks

b) Describe the actions you could take if your spinal block proves inadequate on testing prior to starting surgery for an elective (category 4) caesarean section. 3 marks

c) What are the early symptoms and signs of a spinal block that is ascending too high? 5 marks

d) How should you manage a patient who complains of pain during an elective caesarean section under spinal anaesthesia? 6 marks

Q4 — Intrauterine foetal death

A woman, who has had an intrauterine foetal death (IUFD) at 36 weeks' gestation in her first pregnancy, is admitted to the delivery suite for induction of labour.

a) List the causes of IUFD. 4 marks

b) Describe the important non-clinical aspects of her management. 3 marks

c) What are the considerations when providing pain relief for this woman prior to delivery? 5 marks

d) What are the options for pain relief? 4 marks

e) If this patient requires a caesarean section what are the advantages of using regional anaesthesia, other than the avoidance of the effects of general anaesthesia? 4 marks

Q5 — Obesity and pregnancy

A primiparous patient with a BMI of 55kg/m^2 presents in the high-risk anaesthetic antenatal assessment clinic at 34 weeks' gestation. She is hoping to have a normal delivery.

a) What are the specific cardiorespiratory effects of obesity in the pregnant patient? 4 marks

b) What are the specific obstetric concerns associated with a raised BMI in pregnancy? 3 marks

c) What are the foetal risks associated with a high BMI? 3 marks

d) What are your anaesthetic concerns in this obstetric patient with a high BMI? 6 marks

e) What are your considerations when you provide labour analgesia? 4 marks

Q6 — Surgery in pregnancy

A 28-year-old woman presents for an acute appendicectomy under general anaesthesia; she is 22 weeks pregnant.

a) List the risks to the foetus during anaesthesia in this situation. 4 marks

b) How can the risks to the foetus be minimised? 2 marks

c) How does timing the surgery reduce the foetal risk? 1 mark

d) What steps would you take to avoid foetal hypoxia? 5 marks

e) List any four drugs used in anaesthetic practice and their adverse effects on the foetus. 4 marks

f) What additional preoperative and intraoperative steps would you take to ensure foetal safety if she is 27 weeks pregnant instead? 4 marks

Q7 — Airway problems in pregnancy

a) What factors may contribute to difficulties encountered when securing the airway under general anaesthesia in the pregnant patient? 9 marks

b) What measures can be taken to reduce airway-related morbidity and mortality associated with general anaesthesia in a pregnant woman? 8 marks

c) What are the recommendations in the 4th National Audit Project (Major Complications of Airway Management in the UK, NAP4) regarding airway management in the pregnant woman? 3 marks

Q8 — Mitral stenosis in pregnancy

A 27-year-old woman is 13 weeks pregnant. In the antenatal clinic she is found to have an asymptomatic heart murmur. A subsequent echocardiogram shows moderate to severe mitral stenosis.

a) List the causes of mitral stenosis (MS). 2 marks

b) What are the echocardiographic criteria for the diagnosis of severity of MS? 2 marks

c) What is the normal mitral valve area and at what point does the patient become symptomatic with MS? 2 marks

d) What are the cardiovascular changes in pregnancy that could exacerbate the pathophysiology of MS? 3 marks

e) How do the cardiovascular changes in pregnancy exacerbate the pathophysiology of MS? 3 marks

f) What are your cardiovascular goals when she presents in labour? 2 marks

g) Outline your management of this patient in labour. 5 marks

h) Explain the mechanism of pulmonary oedema post-delivery. 1 mark

Q9 — Amniotic fluid embolism

A 39-year-old multiparous woman is admitted post-term with spontaneous rupture of membranes and meconium-stained liquor. After an epidural catheter is inserted, a syntocinon infusion is started as she is in early labour. She started contracting shortly and the foetal heart rate drops. She becomes breathless and cyanosed; her blood pressure has dropped.

a) What are the differential diagnoses for this presentation? 6 marks

b) What are the risk factors for an amniotic fluid embolism (AFE)? 2 marks

c) Describe the pathogenesis of AFE. 2 marks

d) What are the clinical features of AFE? 4 marks

e) How would you diagnose AFE? 2 marks

f) What is the incidence of AFE? 1 mark

g) List the management strategies for AFE. 3 marks

Q10 — Labour analgesia and puerperal sepsis

a) Describe the pain pathways associated with the first and second stages of labour. 2 marks

b) Explain how and why the nature of the pain experienced changes as labour progresses. 2 marks

c) What dermatomes should be blocked for labour analgesia and a lower segment caesarean section (LSCS)? 2 marks

d) Why is it essential to achieve a higher dermatomal level of regional block for a caesarean section than for analgesia in labour? 1 mark

e) Why do you sometimes observe bradycardia during regional anaesthesia for a caesarean section? 2 marks

f) List any five specific situations in which labour epidurals may be beneficial. 4 marks

g) What is puerperal sepsis? 2 marks

h) Name the organisms implicated in sepsis in the UK. 2 marks

i) List the risk factors for sepsis. 3 marks

Chapter 3

Paediatric anaesthesia

QUESTIONS

Q1 — Down's syndrome

A 9-year-old child is listed for a dental extraction in a day-case list.

a) List the cardiovascular problems in Down's syndrome relevant to an anaesthetist. 2 marks

b) List the airway/respiratory problems in Down's syndrome of relevance to the anaesthetist. 5 marks

c) List the neurological problems that are associated with this syndrome in children and its relevance to the anaesthetist. 3 marks

d) What are the potential problems during induction of anaesthesia and the initial airway management in this patient? 6 marks

e) What are the possible specific difficulties in the postoperative management of this child? 4 marks

Q2 — Day-case eye surgery

A 4-year-old boy is listed for elective strabismus surgery in a day-case ophthalmology theatre list.

a) List the anaesthetic considerations for this patient with regards to his age. 4 marks

b) List the anaesthetic considerations of this case with regards to day-case surgery. 3 marks

c) List the anaesthetic considerations with regards to strabismus surgery. 4 marks

d) During the operation, the patient suddenly develops a profound bradycardia. What is your immediate management of this situation? 2 marks

e) What strategies would you employ to reduce postoperative nausea and vomiting (PONV) in this patient? 4 marks

f) What strategies would you employ to reduce postoperative pain in this child? 3 marks

Q3 — Meningococcal sepsis

You are called to the emergency department to see a 2-year-old child who presents with a 4-hour history of high temperature and drowsiness. On examination, there is a prolonged capillary refill time and a non-blanching rash. A presumptive diagnosis of meningococcal septicaemia is made.

a) What is the normal weight, pulse rate, systolic arterial blood pressure and capillary refill time for a child of this age? 4 marks

b) Define appropriate resuscitation goals for this child. 2 marks

c) Outline the management in the first 15 minutes after presentation. 6 marks

d) After 15 minutes, the child remains shocked and is unresponsive to fluid. What is the most likely pathophysiological derangement in this child's circulation? 2 marks

e) What are the important further treatment options in this case after the first 15 to 20 minutes? 6 marks

Q4 — Hernia repair in preterm babies

A 12-week-old male baby presents for a unilateral inguinal hernia repair. He was born at 30 weeks' gestation (30/40).

a) What are the airway and respiratory concerns in this baby? 5 marks

b) What are the circulatory and metabolic concerns in this patient? 5 marks

c) What oxygen saturation range would you aim to achieve in this patient and why? 2 marks

d) List four other possible major morbidities that could be associated in this child. 2 marks

e) What are the advantages of general anaesthesia for this baby? 3 marks

f) What are the disadvantages of general anaesthesia for this baby? 3 marks

Q5 — Upper respiratory infection and anaesthesia

A 5-year-old boy presents for a myringotomy and grommet insertion as a day case. During your preoperative assessment you notice that he has nasal discharge.

a) Why would it be inappropriate to cancel the operation with this information? 1 mark

b) What are the potential anaesthetic problems in a child with upper respiratory tract infection? 4 marks

c) List five features in the history that would potentially cause an increased risk of airway complications. 5 marks

d) List five features in the examination that would potentially cause an increased risk of airway complications. 5 marks

e) What perioperative airway factors would you consider in decision-making? 2 marks

f) What social factors would prevent this child being treated as a day case? 3 marks

Q6 — Foreign body inhalation in a child

An 8-year-old girl is suspected to have inhaled a plastic bead while playing. She looks frightened, is coughing, has an audible stridor and is saturating 96% on room air.

a) List any three possible complications from foreign body inhalation. 3 marks

b) What are the main features in the preoperative assessment of a child who has an inhaled foreign body? 5 marks

c) What are the main challenges during surgery for foreign body retrieval from the airway? 4 marks

d) What are the key goals of intraoperative anaesthetic conduct? 6 marks

e) What postoperative measures could help in a suspected traumatic bronchoscopy? 2 marks

Q7 — Congenital diaphragmatic hernia

A 31-year-old primiparous lady had an emergency caesarean section for foetal distress. You are the anaesthetist and deliver her by general anaesthesia. The paediatrician calls you for help as the delivered baby has respiratory distress. This neonate is later diagnosed with a congenital diaphragmatic hernia.

a) Name four other causes of respiratory distress in a newborn. 4 marks

b) What is the aetiology for a congenital diaphragmatic hernia? 2 marks

c) Name a few other conditions that are associated with a congenital diaphragmatic hernia. 2 marks

d) Name any two factors of severity that worsen the outcome and increase mortality. 2 marks

e) Based on embryology, what are the two types of congenital diaphragmatic hernia? 1 mark

f) What are the medical treatments for congenital diaphragmatic hernia and how would you optimise the patient before the surgery? 5 marks

g) This neonate mentioned above was taken to the operating theatre for emergency open surgery and repair after stabilisation; what are the intraoperative challenges in this neonate? 4 marks

Q8 — Non-accidental injury

A 4-year-old girl is admitted to the accident and emergency department and the staff has raised the suspicion of a non-accidental injury.

a) What types of physical injury would raise concerns of abuse in a child of this age? 4 marks

b) What timely action must be taken as a result of your concerns? 7 marks

c) List the parental factors that are known to increase the risk of child abuse. 5 marks

d) List the features of a child's past medical history that are known to increase the risk of child abuse. 2 marks

e) List the modes of presentation in the case of child neglect. 2 marks

Q9 — Epiglottitis

A 3-year-old child presents to the accident and emergency department with a short history of respiratory distress, fever, drooling and stridor.

a) List the differential diagnoses for this child's condition. 5 marks

b) What is the causative organism for epiglottitis? 1 mark

c) How would you initially manage this child? 6 marks

d) List the advantages of inhalational induction in this child. 4 marks

e) List the potential advantages of intravenous induction in this child. 4 marks

Q10 — Palliative care in a child

A 6-year-old child is diagnosed to have severe spastic quadriplegic cerebral palsy. This boy is wheelchair-bound, has a gastrostomy, needs frequent suctioning due to excess secretions in the respiratory tract, and suffers with epileptic fits. In his recent intensive care admission, his respiratory failure is severe and his clinical condition deteriorates.

a) What are the priniciples of paediatric palliative care in general? 3 marks

b) Name a few standards of care in paediatric palliative care, based on the Together for Short Lives Core Care Pathway for children with life-limiting and life-threatening conditions. 6 marks

c) What are the factors to consider in pain management in this child and what management strategies would you use? 4 marks

d) What are the factors to consider if this child has agitation and how would you manage it? 4 marks

e) If this child has nausea and vomiting, how would you manage this? 3 marks

Q11 — Endoscopy in a child

An 8-year-old girl is listed for an upper and lower GI endoscopy on a gastroenterology list.

a) List a few conditions that would need endoscopy in a child of this age. 4 marks

b) How would you assess this child for anaesthetic need for the endoscopy? 3 marks

c) Name a few anaesthetic techniques that could be used in this patient and describe how you would do them. 6 marks

d) What post-procedure care is needed after the endoscopy is done in this child? 3 marks

e) List any four indications for tracheal intubation for endoscopic procedures in children. 4 marks

Q12 — Pyloric stenosis

A 3-week-old preterm baby is admitted with complaints of projectile vomiting of non-bilious stomach contents and dehydration. A provisional diagnosis of hypertrophic obstructive pyloric stenosis is made by the paediatric team.

a) What is the aetiology of pyloric stenosis? 2 marks

b) What are the electrolyte changes that can occur in this patient and what is the mechanism for these changes? 6 marks

c) If the electrolyte changes are not corrected, can you take this patient to the operating theatre as an emergency to correct the stenosis? 2 marks

d) What are the surgical options in pyloric stenois? 2 marks

e) What are the anaesthetic considerations for this child with pyloric stenosis? 6 marks

f) What are the analgesic techniques that you could use in this patient? 2 marks

Chapter 4

Pain
QUESTIONS

Q1 — Persistent postoperative pain

a) Define persistent postoperative pain. 3 marks

b) List five surgical procedures that are most commonly associated with persistent postoperative pain. 5 marks

c) What are the risk factors for the development of persistent postoperative pain? 8 marks

d) What pathophysiological changes occur at the spinal cord level during the transition from acute to persistent postoperative pain? 4 marks

Q2 — Opioids, spinal cord stimulators and intrathecal pumps

a) How should you manage the perioperative opioid requirements of a patient who is having elective surgery and who takes regular opioids for non-malignant pain? 8 marks

b) Give the conversion factors for oral tramadol, codeine and oxycodone to the equianalgesic oral morphine dose. 3 marks

c) What are the perioperative implications of an existing spinal cord stimulator? 6 marks

d) What additional perioperative precautions should be taken if the patient has an intrathecal drug delivery system fitted? 3 marks

Q3 — Neuropathic pain

a) What is neuropathic pain? 2 marks

b) List a few pain descriptors used by patients to describe their neuropathic pain. 2 marks

c) List any four examples of neuropathic pain. 2 marks

d) List any three commonly used medications to manage neuropathic pain and explain their mechanism of action. 6 marks

e) What pain scales are used to assess neuropathic pain? 2 marks

f) Give examples of unidimensional pain scales. 3 marks

g) Give examples of multidimensional pain scales. 2 marks

h) List any two pain assessment tools that you would use in a 5-year-old child after an appendicectomy in the immediate postoperative period. 1 mark

Q4 — Complex regional pain syndrome

A 37-year-old female is referred to the pain clinic with a possible diagnosis of complex regional pain syndrome (CRPS). She had a right wrist fracture and was in a plaster cast for 6 weeks. She developed severe pain even on light touch as soon as the cast was removed.

a) What is CRPS? 2 marks

b) How is CRPS classified? 1 mark

c) List the symptoms and signs of CRPS from the Budapest diagnostic criteria and explain these criteria. 8 marks

d) How would you manage and treat this patient with CRPS? 9 marks

Q5 — Pain relief in cancer

You are asked to review a patient with advanced cancer on the medical ward for pain relief options.

a) List the causes of pain in a patient with advanced cancer. 5 marks

b) How can side effects from opioid medications be minimised in these patients? 4 marks

c) List the steps in the WHO analgesic ladder for cancer pain. 6 marks

d) What is the most commonly used class of drug used for the management of cancer pain and in what manner are they used to optimise their effect? 2 marks

e) Give three examples of interventional strategies, along with their indications, done by pain specialists to manage cancer pain. 3 marks

Q6 — Problems due to opioids

A 48-year-old male attends the pre-anaesthetic clinic with a chronic use of high-dose opioids for low back pain.

a) Enumerate the long-term side effects and concerns with opioids if used for non-cancer pain. 6 marks

b) Define tolerance, physical dependence and addiction. 3 marks

c) What is opioid-induced hyperalgesia (OIH)? 2 marks

d) What are the presenting features of OIH? 2 marks

e) How would you manage a patient with OIH? 2 marks

f) What would be your substitute drug with the aim of reducing opioids in this patient in a pain clinic? 2 marks

g) What are the aims and principles of substitution therapy in such patients? 3 marks

Q7 — Intrathecal opioids

a) What are the sites of action of intrathecal (IT) opioids? 2 marks

b) What are the intracellular and extracellular mechanisms of analgesic effect within the spinal cord following the administration of IT opioids? 6 marks

c) List the principal side effects of IT opioids. 4 marks

d) List the factors that may increase the risk of postoperative respiratory depression following the administration of IT opioids. 5 marks

e) What is the role of antihistamines in opioid-induced pruritis? 2 marks

f) How would you manage opioid-induced pruritis? 1 mark

Q8 — Phantom limb pain

You are called to see a 74-year-old male patient who has had a below-knee amputation 24 hours ago. Despite using a patient-controlled analgesia (PCA) pump with intravenous morphine, he is still in severe pain.

a) Mention the possible causes/reasons for inadequate pain control in this patient. 4 marks

b) How would you optimise perioperative pain control in a patient having an amputation of a lower limb? 6 marks

c) List the types of post-amputation pain that patients may present with. 3 marks

d) List the features of post-amputation pain syndrome (phantom limb pain). 3 marks

e) Enumerate the pharmacological options available for managing post-amputation pain syndrome. 4 marks

Q9 — Pain with fractured ribs

You are called to the emergency department to assess a 70-year-old man with known chronic obstructive pulmonary disease (COPD). He has sustained fractures to his 8th, 9th and 10th ribs due to a fall. He has no other injuries. He is currently on paracetamol and codeine which are not helping him with his pain relief.

a) List the possible respiratory effects of inadequate analgesia from fractured ribs. 3 mark

b) What are the secondary respiratory complications resulting from fractured ribs? 1 mark

c) List the key management strategies in optimising the ventilation in a patient with fractured ribs. 4 mark

d) What is the purpose of a rib fracture score? 2 mark

e) How would you assess the adequacy of pain relief in this patient? 3 mark

f) What are the measures used to manage analgesia following fractured ribs? 7 mark

Q10 — Back pain

a) List the causes of mechanical (musculoskeletal) back pain. 3 mark

b) List five examples of red flags whilst assessing a patient for back pain. 5 mark

c) List three causes of nerve root pain. 3 mark

d) What is the recommendation for paracetamol in managing mechanical back pain as per the NICE guidelines? 1 mark

e) What is the recommendation for opioids in chronic low back pain as per the NICE guidelines? 1 mark

f) What is the role of epidural injections in low back pain as per the NICE guidelines? 2 marks

g) When should you perform radiofrequency denervation of the median branch nerve in a case of chronic back pain? 1 mark

h) List the non-invasive interventions for low back pain and sciatica. 4 marks

Q11 — Trigeminal neuralgia

a) List any five characteristic features of trigeminal neuralgia. 5 marks

b) What are the pathophysiological causes of trigeminal neuralgia? 3 marks

c) List any one cause of non-idiopathic secondary trigeminal neuralgia. 1 mark

d) What investigations might help in the diagnosis of secondary trigeminal neuralgia? 1 mark

e) What is the first-line management for trigeminal neuralgia and give some examples? 3 marks

f) What are the possible side effects with carbamazepine? 3 marks

g) What are the interventional management options for trigeminal neuralgia? 4 mark

Q12 — Post-herpetic neuralgia

A 57-year-old female had shingles 2 years ago in her right T8 dermatome and has suffered with severe pain in that dermatome since then. Her sleep and mood are significantly affected.

a) What is post-herpetic neuralgia? 1 mark

b) What is the cause of *Herpes zoster*? 2 mark

c) Describe the pathophysiology of pain in post-herpetic neuralgia. 4 mark

d) List any six risk factors for post-herpetic neuralgia. 3 mark

e) How would you prevent post-herpetic neuralgia? 3 mark

f) How would you treat post-herpetic neuralgia? 7 mark

Chapter 5

Cardiac anaesthesia

QUESTIONS

Q1 — CABG complications

a) What are the central and peripheral neurological complications of coronary artery bypass surgery? **3 marks**

b) List any five risk factors for central neurological complications in these surgeries. **5 marks**

c) What are the pathophysiologic mechanisms involved in the neurologic complications after these surgeries? **4 marks**

d) Name any four intraoperative techniques that are used for monitoring cerebral perfusion during cardiac surgery. **4 marks**

e) List four techniques that could reduce the incidence of central neurological complications. **4 marks**

Q2 — Off-pump bypass

a) List four theoretical advantages of 'off-pump' coronary artery bypass (OPCAB) grafting compared with an 'on-bypass' technique. **4 marks**

b) What are the four potential mechanisms of haemodynamic instability during OPCAB grafting? 4 mark

c) List any three anaesthetic strategies that help to minimise this haemodynamic instability. 6 mark

d) List three important mechanisms to maintain coronary perfusion during off-pump CABG. 3 mark

e) What are the potential disadvantages of OPCAB grafting? 3 mark

Q3 — Cardiac tamponade

You are asked to review a 65-year-old woman on the cardiac intensive care unit who has undergone coronary artery bypass surgery earlier in the day.

a) List any six clinical features that might suggest the development of cardiac tamponade. 8 mark

b) Name four investigations with their findings that could confirm the diagnosis of cardiac tamponade. 6 mark

c) Outline the key steps of acute cardiac tamponade management in this patient. 4 mark

d) Name any two other causes of cardiac tamponade. 2 mark

Q4 — Implantable cardiac devices

a) List any four possible indications for the insertion of a cardiac implantable permanent pacemaker. 4 marks

b) List any four possible indications for the insertion of a cardiac implantable cardioverter defibrillator (ICD). 4 marks

c) What factors would you check/consider preoperatively in a patient with these types of devices? 6 marks

d) Outline the main features of intraoperative and postoperative management of patients with these types of devices having elective surgery under general anaesthetic. 6 marks

Q5 — One-lung ventilation

a) How can the risks associated with lung resection be quantified preoperatively? 6 marks

b) List any six factors that can lead to the development of high airway pressures during one-lung ventilation (OLV). 4 marks

c) How would you manage the development of hypoxaemia during OLV? 8 marks

d) What analgesic methods could be used for thoracic surgeries? 2 marks

Q6 — Dilated cardiomyopathy

a) List any three presenting clinical features of dilated cardiomyopathy (DCM). 3 marks

b) What are the pharmacological and non-pharmacological management options for a patient with DCM? 5 marks

c) List the predictors of poor outcome in patients with DCM undergoing surgery. 2 marks

d) What are the haemodynamic goals when anaesthetising patients with DCM? 4 mark

e) What measures would you take to achieve these haemodynamic goals during anaesthesia? 6 mark

Q7 — Aortic stenosis surgery

A 70-year-old woman with aortic stenosis presents for an open aortic valve replacement (AVR).

a) What are the three most common aetiological causes of aortic stenosis? 3 mark

b) What are the main pathophysiological factors responsible for deterioration in a patient with aortic stenosis? 4 marks

c) Which specific symptoms may be used in assessing the progression of this woman's disease and correlate directly with 50% mortality? 3 marks

d) Which specific cardiac investigations would you ask for in assessing this women preoperatively? 3 marks

e) Give values for the peak aortic flow velocity, mean pressure gradient and valve area that would indicate that this woman has severe aortic stenosis. 3 marks

f) What would be your haemodynamic goals for the perioperative management of this patient? 4 marks

Q8 — Lung resection and investigations

A 67-year-old male attends the clinic for a preoperative assessment before a right lower lobe lung resection for a localised non-small cell cancer.

a) Name any three bedside pulmonary function tests that could be done in this patient. 3 marks

b) What are the diagnostic criteria for COPD based on spirometry? 1 mark

c) What does lung carbon monoxide transfer factor (TLCO) indicate and what is its significance? 2 marks

d) What suggestive values of FVC (forced vital capacity) might need mechanical ventilation in neuromuscular diseases? 2 marks

e) What is the NICE guidance on preoperative testing with regards to spirometry in the normal general population? 1 mark

f) In the above question with regards to the patient's lung resection, what is the role of pulmonary function tests (PFTs) and how would you interpret them? 6 marks

g) Name a few techniques of calculating the ppo (predicted postoperative) pulmonary function. 3 marks

h) What are the selection criteria for the suitability of lung volume reduction surgery (LVRS)? 2 marks

Q9 — Cardiac transplantation in children

A 13-year-old child is listed in the cardiac theatre for a heart transplantation for end-stage heart failure.

a) What are the indications for cardiac transplantation in children? 2 marks

b) Name four factors that are important in organ allocation with regards to transplantation. 4 marks

c) What factors would you consider during induction of anaesthesia in this child? 2 marks

d) How would you manage intraoperatively? 2 marks

e) What immunosuppressant therapies are you aware of for induction therapy and maintenance therapy? 2 marks

f) What are the complications that can occur after transplantation? 4 marks

g) If this child has a successful transplant and presents to you for an elective surgery at a later date, what factors would you consider? 4 marks

Q10 — Right ventricular failure

A 69-year-old obese female presents with a significant history of obstructive sleep apnoea with presenting features of right ventricular failure. She has been using a CPAP machine for the last 4 years.

a) What are the signs of acute right ventricular failure? 2 marks

b) What are the signs of chronic right ventricular failure? 2 marks

c) Describe one investigation that will help in the early diagnosis for right ventricular failure. 1 mark

d) Discuss the pathophysiology of right ventricular failure. 4 marks

e) How can obesity lead to right ventricular dysfunction? 2 marks

f) What is the mechanism of right ventricular failure in obstructive sleep apnoea? 2 marks

g) List the management strategies for a patient admitted with right ventricular failure. 7 marks

Chapter 6

Intensive care
QUESTIONS

Q1 — Major haemorrhage

A 45-year-old man has a major haemorrhage following significant trauma and is admitted to the emergency department. He does not have a head injury.

a) Give any two definitions of a major haemorrhage. 2 marks

b) What are the principles of management of a major haemorrhage in this patient? 8 marks

c) List any three metabolic complications that might follow a massive blood transfusion. 3 marks

d) What are the immunologic complications that can occur after a massive blood transfusion? 3 marks

e) What are the other complications that might follow a massive blood transfusion? 4 marks

Q2 — Nutritional support in intensive care

A 45-year-old man with a history of ulcerative colitis and alcohol abuse is admitted to the intensive care unit for inotropic and ventilatory support following a laparotomy to excise a toxic megacolon. His Body Mass Index is 18kg/m^2.

a) Why should this patient receive early nutritional support? 3 marks

b) List any four clinical benefits of early nutrition. 4 marks

c) What are the routes of nutrition and daily energy requirements for this patient? 2 marks

d) What are the basic nutritional requirements in critical illness? 6 marks

e) List two advantages of enteral nutrition. 2 marks

f) List three disadvantages of enteral nutrition. 3 marks

Q3 — Ventilator-associated pneumonia

a) What are the key features in the definition of ventilator-associated pneumonia (VAP)? 3 marks

b) List the risk factors for the development of VAP. 8 marks

c) What measures could be taken to reduce the risk of development of VAP? 8 marks

d) What are bundles of care? 1 mark

Q4 — Acute respiratory distress syndrome

a) List the criteria for a diagnosis of acute respiratory distress syndrome (ARDS). 3 marks

b) How would you classify ARDS? 3 marks

c) List any four clinical indices to quantify oxygenation in ARDS. 4 marks

d) What are the ventilatory strategies in managing a patient with ARDS? 5 marks

e) What are the non-ventilatory strategies in managing a patient with ARDS? 5 marks

Q5 — Sepsis, qSOFA and sepsis bundles

a) Define sepsis and septic shock. 2 marks

b) What are the features of RED FLAG sepsis? 8 marks

c) What are the criteria of the qSOFA (quick SOFA) score? 3 marks

d) How is the qSOFA score useful? 2 marks

e) List the elements of sepsis bundle interventions. 5 marks

Q6 — Transfer of critically ill patients

You are asked to transfer a 43-year-old male patient from an intensive care unit to a specialised neurointensive care unit in a hospital 1 hour away by ambulance.

a) What are the technical risks with regards to the transfer of patients from critical care units? 3 marks

b) What are the non-technical risks that are to be noted during the transfer of critical care patients? 3 marks

c) Describe the organisational risks in the transfer of critically ill patients. 2 marks

d) What guidelines are you aware of regarding the transfer of critically ill patients? 2 marks

e) What would you consider in the process of transfer? 2 marks

f) Describe the essentialities in an ABCDE approach with regard to the transfer of a sick patient. 5 marks

g) List the communication processes that are essential in the transfer of sick patients. 3 marks

Q7 — Propofol-related infusion syndrome

a) What is propofol-related infusion syndrome (PRIS)? 3 marks

b) What are the clinical effects of PRIS? 4 marks

c) List the risk factors for PRIS. 5 marks

d) What specific laboratory findings might be expected in a case of PRIS? 3 marks

e) How may PRIS be prevented? 3 marks

f) How would you manage PRIS? 2 marks

Q8 — Guillain-Barré syndrome

A 68-year-old man is referred to the neurointensive care unit with suspected Guillain-Barré syndrome.

a) What is Guillain-Barré syndrome (GBS) and what are its causes? 5 marks

b) List the clinical features of GBS. 5 marks

c) List the investigations/findings that can be used to aid the diagnosis. 6 marks

d) What supportive treatment is needed in this patient with GBS? 2 marks

e) What specific therapies are available for GBS? 2 marks

Q9 — Renal replacement therapy

a) What are the renal indications for starting renal replacement therapy (RRT) in the intensive care setting (ICU)? 4 marks

b) What are the non-renal indications for starting RRT in the ICU? 4 marks

c) List the types of RRT available in intensive care. 6 marks

d) Outline the principal mechanisms of solute and water removal by filtration. 3 marks

e) Outline the principles of haemodialysis. 3 marks

Q10 — Refeeding syndrome

a) What is the daily energy requirement of a normal healthy 70kg man? **1 mark**

b) What are the recommended daily proportions of carbohydrate, fat and protein? **3 marks**

c) What is refeeding syndrome? **2 marks**

d) What are the three major electrolyte abnormalities seen in refeeding syndrome? **3 marks**

e) What is the commonest electrolyte nutritional deficiency? **1 mark**

f) Which patients are at particular risk of refeeding syndrome? **6 marks**

g) How should the nutritional requirements of those 'at risk' be managed? **4 marks**

Q11 — Intra-abdominal hypertension

A 52-year-old male is admitted to the intensive care unit with a provisional diagnosis of intra-abdominal hypertension and oliguria.

a) Define intra-abdominal hypertension (IAH) and abdominal compartment syndrome. **2 marks**

b) Name any four causes of IAH. **4 marks**

c) What are the pathophysiological consequences of abdominal compartment syndrome? **4 marks**

d) How would you grade the severity of the IAH? 4 marks

e) What techniques could be used to measure intra-abdominal pressure? 2 marks

f) How would you manage the IAH in this patient? 4 marks

Q12 — Stroke and thrombolysis

a) What imaging modalities are recommended by NICE in acute stroke? 2 marks

b) What specific treatments can be considered for acute thrombotic ischaemic strokes? 3 marks

c) What are the other general and supportive treatment measures that you would implement in the treatment of an acute stroke? 3 marks

d) In these patients, what is the potential consequence of severe hypertension? 1 mark

e) What level of hypertension (systolic and diastolic) is regarded as severe after an ischaemic stroke? 2 marks

f) What is the recommendation for arterial BP values in patients for thrombolysis? 1 mark

g) A patient has had a large hemispheric infarction following a stroke. Outline your management of this patient following admission to critical care. 8 marks

Q13 — Diabetic ketoacidosis

You are asked to review an 18-year-old male in the emergency department who has been found obtunded at home. He is an insulin-dependent diabetic with a history of poor control. Capillary blood glucose is 23.4mmol/L.

a) List the biochemical findings that confirm the diagnosis of diabetic ketoacidosis (DKA). 2 marks

b) What are the clinical features of DKA? List at least two signs and two symptoms. 2 marks

c) What other clinical and biochemical findings are seen in severe DKA? 2 marks

d) What is the pathophysiology of DKA? 1 mark

e) What are the three most common causes of DKA? 3 marks

f) What investigations would you request in such a presentation of DKA? 3 marks

g) Outline the management plan for severe DKA within the first hour. 4 marks

h) What are the serious complications that can follow the management of DKA? 1 mark

i) What is the mechanism of hypokalaemia in DKA and how is it managed? 2 marks

Q14 — Scoring systems, NEWS and ICNARC

Scoring systems are routinely used in intensive care units for critically ill patients.

a) What is a scoring system? 1 mark

b) What types of scoring systems are you aware of in critical care patients? 2 marks

c) Describe the commonly used score in your intensive care unit and explain how you would use it. 2 marks

d) Why are early warning scores useful in acute illness and sepsis? 2 marks

e) Give some examples of early intervention that could be offered if the early warning scores indicate the need. 2 marks

f) List the advantages and limits of early warning scores. 2 marks

g) List the features used in the National Early Warning Score (NEWS). 3 marks

h) What are the ICNARC reports? 2 marks

i) What are the limitations of the ICNARC reports? 4 marks

Q15 — Long-term venous access

a) What are the main indications for long-term venous access? 3 marks

b) What are the common types of long-term venous catheters? 4 marks

c) What are the main considerations for choosing the insertion site for long-term venous access? 4 marks

d) What is the ideal site for catheter tip position? 4 marks

e) What are the complications of long-term venous catheters? 5 marks

Q16 — ICU-acquired weakness

a) What are the main types of intensive care unit (ICU)-acquired weakness? 3 marks

b) What are the risk factors for ICU-acquired weakness? 4 marks

c) What are the main postulated mechanisms in the development of ICU-acquired weakness? 4 marks

d) What are the main clinical features essential for diagnosing ICU-acquired weakness? 5 marks

e) What are the main complications associated with ICU-acquired weakness? 2 marks

f) What is the mainstay of treatment of ICU-acquired weakness? 2 marks

Chapter 7

Perioperative medicine

QUESTIONS

Q1 — Thyroidectomy

A patient presents for a total thyroidectomy.

a) Name any five specific investigations that are indicated in the preoperative assessment and explain why they are indicated. 5 marks

b) What factors in a euthyroid patient must the anaesthetist consider during the induction and maintenance phases of a total thyroidectomy? 7 marks

c) During extubation, what factors must be considered post-total thyroidectomy? 4 marks

d) List any four important postoperative complications following this surgery and how you would manage them. 4 marks

Q2 — Diabetes and anaesthesia

You are assessing a 63-year-old female for an elective laparotomy in the pre-anaesthetic assessment clinic. She has type I diabetes which is under control.

a) In a patient with diabetes mellitus, what clinical features may indicate autonomic involvement? 4 marks

b) What are the other microvascular and macrovascular complications of diabetes mellitus? 6 marks

c) List any five classes of oral hypoglycaemic agents that are available with an example. Describe the mechanism of action for each. 10 marks

Q3 — Enhanced recovery programme

A 74-year-old patient is scheduled for a primary total hip replacement.

a) What are the advantages of an enhanced recovery programme (ERP) for this type of surgery? 5 marks

b) What preoperative measures can be included in the ERP for this patient? 5 marks

c) List the intraoperative measures that can be included as part of the ERP in this case. 7 marks

d) What postoperative measures can be included as part of the ERP for this patient? 3 marks

Q4 — Anaemia and anaesthesia

A 76-year-old patient who is scheduled for an elective primary total knee replacement is found to be anaemic, with a haemoglobin level of 90g/L.

a) List the perioperative consequences associated with preoperative anaemia. **5 marks**

b) Name some physiological adaptations that can occur to offset the effects of anaemia. **5 marks**

c) List any five perioperative events that may worsen the effects of anaemia. **5 marks**

d) List further blood tests that may help to classify this anaemia. **5 marks**

Q5 — CPET testing

a) List the main measures of fitness obtained by CPET testing and explain what it is. **4 marks**

b) List any four abnormalities on CPET testing that indicate cardiorespiratory disease with the values. **4 marks**

c) What are the indications for CPET testing? **3 marks**

d) List other tests to assess the patient's functional capacity. **3 marks**

e) What scoring systems can help to predict perioperative risk before major non-cardiac surgery? **6 marks**

Q6 — Prehabilitation

a) What is prehabilitation in perioperative medicine? **1 mark**

b) What are the outcome benefits of a prehabilitation programme? **3 marks**

c) Which specific issues are addressed as part of medical optimisation in a prehabilitation programme? 6 mark

d) How would a prehabilitation exercise program improve a patient's cardiorespiratory reserve? 4 mark

e) What are the benefits of carbohydrate preloading and nutritional optimisation? 4 mark

f) What psychologically supportive interventions may be used in prehabilitation? 2 mark

Q7 — Scoring systems in anaesthesia

a) Describe the risk assessment tools commonly used in anaesthesia. 2 mark

b) Name and describe a risk score for cardiac complications. 2 mark

c) Name and detail a risk score for postoperative pulmonary complications. 2 mark

d) What are the components of the POSSUM and P-POSSUM risk prediction models? 6 mark

e) What is the NELA calculator and what does it estimate? 2 mark

f) The NCEPOD enquiry in 2011 produced the SORT tool; list any four variables that are used in this tool. 2 mark

g) Outline the difference between risk scores and risk prediction models. 4 mark

Chapter 8

Regional, orthopaedic and trauma anaesthesia

QUESTIONS

Q1 — Nerve block for shoulder surgery

a) List the specific nerves that need to be blocked to achieve effective analgesia for shoulder surgery. 6 marks

b) Name any six possible complications of an interscalene block. 6 marks

c) What positioning is needed for shoulder surgery? 1 mark

d) List any three complications of positioning for shoulder surgery. 3 marks

e) What postoperative advice would you give to a patient who has received an interscalene block? 4 marks

Q2 — Regional block in hip fractures

An 80-year-old woman is admitted to hospital having sustained a proximal femoral (neck of femur) fracture in a fall.

a) How would you optimise this patient's pain preoperatively? 5 marks

b) What is the nerve supply of the skin overlying the hip joint? 5 marks

c) What regional nerve blocks can be used to provide preoperative analgesia? 2 marks

d) What nerves are blocked by the fascia iliaca block? 2 marks

e) List the scoring systems that can be used to predict 30-day mortality in this patient. 2 marks

f) List the AAGBI recommendations regarding unacceptable reasons for delaying surgery. 4 marks

Q3 — Ultrasound

a) Outline the basic physical principles involved in the formation of an ultrasound image. 1 mark

b) What is piezoelectrical activity and how is it utilised in ultrasound? 2 marks

c) What governs the reflection of sound waves and the formation of an ultrasound image? 2 marks

d) List the patient factors that influence ultrasound image quality. 4 marks

e) What acoustic artefacts may influence the ultrasound image quality? 4 marks

f) Which two needling techniques are commonly used in ultrasound-guided nerve blocks? 2 marks

g) List the advantages and disadvantages of one of these techniques. 5 marks

Q4 — Spinal cord transection injury

A 19-year-old patient has suffered a complete transection of the spinal cord at the first thoracic vertebral level due to a fall but has no other injuries.

a) What is the pathophysiology of neurological injury subsequent to the fall in this patient? 3 marks

b) What is the cause of neurogenic shock in this patient and how does it present? 1 mark

c) How would spinal shock present in this patient and what are the phases? 2 marks

d) What disturbances may occur subsequently in the cardiovascular system? 4 marks

e) What effects may be seen in the respiratory system? 4 marks

f) When and why may suxamethonium be contraindicated in this patient? 2 marks

g) Give the advantages of a regional anaesthetic technique for a patient having elective lower limb surgery 2 years after a high thoracic spine transection. 4 marks

Q5 — Wrong-side block and never events

a) List the implications for the patient of an inadvertent wrong-sided peripheral nerve block. 5 marks

b) Summarise the recommendations of the "Stop Before You Block" campaign. 5 marks

c) List the factors that have been identified as contributing to the performance of a wrong-side block. 3 marks

d) Define the term "never event". 2 marks

e) List any five drug-related never events. 5 marks

Q6 — Ankle block

A 32-year-old patient is scheduled for hallux valgus surgery.

a) What anaesthetic options are available for anaesthetising this patient? 3 marks

b) List the nerves supplying the ankle joint. 5 marks

c) Describe the origin and sensory innervation from the posterior tibial nerve. 3 marks

d) Describe the origin and sensory innervation from the deep peroneal nerve. 3 marks

e) Describe the origin and sensory innervation from the superficial peroneal nerve. 3 marks

f) List the disadvantages of using an ankle block for this patient. 3 marks

Q7 — Pelvic fractures

You are called to resuscitate a 26-year-old male who had a major accident while driving a motorcycle. He is diagnosed with a pelvic fracture.

a) How would you classify pelvic fractures? 4 marks

b) How would you initially manage and resuscitate this patient? 6 marks

c) How would you apply a pelvic binder in this patient and how long would you leave it? 2 marks

d) What are the surgical options that are available in this patient? 2 marks

e) What are the anaesthetic considerations in this patient with a traumatic pelvic fracture? 6 marks

Q8 — Bone cement syndrome

A 78-year-old patient is undergoing an elective total hip replacement.

a) During the surgery, when can the patient present with bone cement implantation syndrome (BCIS)? 3 marks

b) What clinical features would make you suspect a BCIS? 1 mark

c) How would you grade the severity of BCIS? 3 marks

d) What is the pathophysiology of BCIS? 4 marks

e) What are the risk factors for the development of BCIS? 5 marks

f) How can surgeons minimise the risk of development of BCIS? 4 marks

Q9 — Nerve injury after a regional block

You are part of the in-patient pain ward round. You are asked by ward staff to review a 38-year-old female who had a femoral nerve block followed by general anaesthesia for an external fixator of her lower leg 2 days ago. She complains of symptoms related to nerve injury in the particular dermatome since the nerve block.

a) What is the incidence of peripheral nerve injury after surgery? 1 mark

b) Explain the anatomy of peripheral nerves in general. 3 marks

c) How would you classify the severity of nerve injury? 2 marks

d) What are the mechanisms of nerve injury? 2 marks

e) What factors would you consider to reduce nerve injury in your practice? 4 marks

f) How would you evaluate the above patient and what diagnostic tests could be used? 2 marks

g) How would you manage this patient? Explain the RA-UK guidelines where appropriate in this management plan. 6 marks

Q10 — Local anaesthetic toxicity

a) What are the clinical features of local anaesthetic systemic toxicity (LAST)? 4 marks

b) What are the mechanisms of LAST? 2 marks

c) What are the risk factors for LAST? 6 marks

d) List a few steps that you could take to prevent LAST. 2 marks

e) How would you manage LAST once it has occurred? 4 marks

f) What are the mechanisms of action of intravenous lipids in LAST? 2 marks

Chapter 9

Other topics in general medicine

QUESTIONS

Q1 — Mental Capacity Act

a) What are the principles underlying the Mental Capacity Act (MCA) 2005? 5 marks

b) How would you define "capacity" with regards to the above act? 2 marks

c) How would you assess capacity? 4 marks

d) What has changed in the consent process since the Montgomery's case? 4 marks

e) Who is responsible for consent? 3 marks

f) If you treat a patient without consent, what could be the consequences? 1 mark

g) Which medical body has laid down the guidance on the consenting process in the UK and cite this guidance? 1 mark

Q2 — Accidental awareness

a) What is accidental awareness under general anaesthesia (AAGA)? 1 mark

b) What is the overall incidence of awareness under general anaesthesia and the estimated awareness incidence for a caesarean section under general anaesthesia as per the NAP5 study? 2 marks

c) List the monitoring devices that can be used to help reduce the incidence of awareness under general anaesthesia. 2 marks

d) What are the factors contributing to the increased incidence of awareness? 10 marks

e) How would you minimise the chances of awareness in anaesthesia? 5 marks

Q3 — NAP6 report on anaphylaxis

a) List the four common triggers for perioperative anaphylaxis according to the report of the National Audit Project 6 (NAP6) from the Royal College of Anaesthetists. 4 marks

b) What is the estimated incidence of perioperative anaphylaxis? 1 mark

c) Outline the pathophysiological process of anaphylaxis. 5 marks

d) Describe your management of intraoperative anaphylaxis in an adult patient. 8 marks

e) What should be done after successful treatment of anaphylaxis? 2 marks

Q4 — Emergency laparotomy and NELA

An 82-year-old male is listed on the emergency operating theatre list for an urgent laparotomy. He presented with an acute abdomen and pain.

a) What is the 30-day mortality for a patient having an emergency laparotomy? 1 mark

b) What are the common indications for an emergency laparotomy as per the National Emergency Laparotomy Audit (NELA) 2015? 2 marks

c) How would you prepare this patient for anaesthesia? 2 marks

d) How would you anaesthetise this patient for an emergency laparotomy? 2 marks

e) List the postoperative considerations in this patient. 2 marks

f) As per the third National Emergency Laparotomy Audit (NELA) 2017, what are the nine key standards of care? 6 marks

g) What are the constituents of the Emergency Laparotomy Pathway Quality Improvement Care (ELPQuiC) bundle? 5 marks

Q5 — Aspiration of gastric contents

A 60-year-old man is having an elective knee arthroscopy and has just aspirated a significant amount of gastric fluid during anaesthesia. He has a supraglottic airway device in place and is breathing spontaneously. His inspired oxygen fraction is 1.0 and the pulse oximeter shows an oxygen saturation of 91%.

a) Describe your immediate management of this patient. 4 mark

b) List the respiratory complications he could develop in the next 48 hours. 2 mark

c) What are the possible preoperative risk factors for regurgitation and aspiration of gastric contents in this case? 4 mark

d) What are the normal physiological mechanisms preventing reflux? 2 mark

e) Describe the strategies available to reduce the risk and impact of aspiration of gastric contents in any patient. 5 mark

f) List the summary of recommendations from NAP4 on aspiration. 3 mark

Q6 — Phaeochromocytoma

A 45-year-old patient is reviewed in the preoperative assessment clinic prior to surgery to excise a phaeochromocytoma.

a) What are the characteristic clinical features of a phaeochromocytoma? 6 mark

b) Which specific biochemical investigations might confirm the diagnosis of a phaeochromocytoma? 2 mark

c) Which specific radiological investigations might confirm the diagnosis of a phaeochromocytoma? 2 marks

d) How would you pharmacologically optimise the cardiovascular system prior to surgery? 6 marks

e) How would you assess the adequacy of cardiovascular optimisation preoperatively? 1 mark

f) Mention the steps in the management of intraoperative hypotension following tumour devascularisation. 3 marks

Q7 — TIVA and TCI

a) What are the indications for total intravenous anaesthesia (TIVA)? 5 marks

b) What are the main components of a target-controlled infusion (TCI) system? 3 marks

c) What are the potential patient problems with TIVA? 2 marks

d) How might each of these problems in question c be minimised? 6 marks

e) What are the potential technical problems with TIVA? 4 marks

Q8 — Obstructive sleep apnoea and STOP-BANG

A patient with obstructive sleep apnoea (OSA) but no other cardiovascular or respiratory comorbidity is scheduled to have peripheral surgery with at least one night stay in the hospital.

a) List all the elements of the STOP-BANG assessment for a patient with suspected OSA. 4 mark

b) How is the STOP-BANG assessment used to quantify risk? 3 mark

c) What are the cardiovascular consequences of OSA? 3 mark

d) What steps can be taken to minimise perioperative risk in this patient having peripheral surgery? 10 mar

Q9 — Postoperative nausea and vomiting

a) List the patient-related risk factors for postoperative nausea and vomiting (PONV). 7 mark

b) What are the anaesthetic related risk factors for PONV in adult patients? 3 mark

c) What are the unwanted effects of PONV in adults? 6 mark

d) Which non-pharmacological interventions have been shown to be effective in reducing PONV in adults? 2 mark

e) Briefly explain the proposed mechanisms of action of 5-HT3 antagonists such as ondansetron when used as an antiemetic. 2 mark

Q10 — Extubation problems

a) List the airway risk factors that may indicate a difficult extubation. 3 mark

b) List the patient factors that you can optimise prior to extubation. 4 marks

c) What other factors can you optimise prior to extubation? 4 marks

d) Enumerate the strategies that you would employ to manage a high-risk extubation. 5 marks

e) Outline the steps you would take to exchange an endotracheal tube for a supraglottic airway device (SAD) to aid extubation. 4 marks

Q11 — LASER and laryngeal surgery

A 77-year-old man is scheduled for laser surgery on a laryngeal tumour.

a) What does the term "LASER" stand for? 1 mark

b) What is the character of the light that forms a LASER? 1 mark

c) What different types of laser can be used for surgery? 3 marks

d) How can the risk of an airway fire be minimised? 5 marks

e) What measures would you take to protect the staff when a laser is in use? 4 marks

f) What anaesthetic techniques can be used to allow a tubeless field for laryngeal surgery? 5 marks

g) Give one example of LASER-resistant endotracheal tubes used in airway surgeries. 1 mark

Q12 — Cerebral palsy

An 8-year-old child is scheduled for an elective right femoral osteotomy due to impending dislocation of the hip. She has severe cerebral palsy.

a) What is cerebral palsy? 3 marks

b) List the causes of cerebral palsy. 3 marks

c) List the typical clinical features of severe cerebral palsy, with its associated anaesthetic implications. Do this for the central nervous system, respiratory system, musculoskeletal system and gastrointestinal system. 8 marks

d) What are the expected problems in providing adequate postoperative analgesia in this patient? 2 marks

e) Outline a management plan to optimise analgesia in this patient. 4 marks

Q13 — Acute pancreatitis

a) List two common causes of acute pancreatitis in the United Kingdom. 1 mark

b) What are the components of the revised Atlanta criteria 2012 for the diagnosis of pancreatitis? 3 marks

c) Classify acute pancreatitis according to the severity. 3 marks

d) What is the role of antibiotics in acute pancreatitis? 2 marks

e) What are the specific principles of managing severe acute pancreatitis in a critical care environment? 7 marks

f) What is the role of surgery and intervention in acute pancreatitis? 4 marks

Q14 — Postoperative pulmonary complications

a) List the postoperative pulmonary complications that may occur following non-cardiothoracic surgery. 3 marks

b) What are the patient-related (4 marks) and surgery-related (2 marks) risk factors for postoperative pulmonary complications following non-cardiothoracic surgery? 6 marks

c) How might anaesthesia contribute to postoperative pulmonary complications? 3 marks

d) What perioperative strategies may you adopt to reduce postoperative pulmonary complications? 5 marks

e) List five lung expansion techniques that could be used postoperatively. 3 marks

Q15 — Drug approval and levels of evidence

a) What is the process of drug approval and what are the types of studies that must be done for drug approval? 5 marks

b) How would you design a study to compare morphine with a newer synthetic opioid in managing pain? 5 marks

c) How would you evaluate the level of evidence available for a treatment? 5 marks

d) How would you stratify the strength of recommendation based on the level of evidence? 5 marks

Q16 — Oxygenation, lateral decubitus and the alveolar gas equation

a) Name four reasons and explain why anaesthetised patients need more than 21% oxygen. 8 marks

b) A patient is listed for lateral decubitus surgery; how does the V/Q ratio alter in dependent and non-dependent lung regions in different positions with anaesthesia and controlled ventilation? 5 marks

c) A 48-year-old female is listed for a laparoscopic cholecystectomy. The monitor shows increased $etCO_2$ with signs of hypercapnia. What is the alveolar gas equation and explain how any increase in alveolar PCO_2 will reduce PO_2 in this patient? 7 marks

Q17 — Effects of smoking

a) What are the clinical effects of cigarette smoking in the following systems? 4 marks

Cardiovascular system: ______________________________

Respiratory system: ______________________________

Gastrointestinal system: ______________________________

Other systems: ____________________

b) Name four constituents of cigarette smoking that cause damage and their common biological effects in the following. 2 marks

Polycyclic hydrocarbons: ____________________

Nitrosamines: ____________________

Aza-arenes: ____________________

Aromatic amines: ____________________

c) How would you describe the affinity of carbon monoxide for haemoglobin compared with that of oxygen? 1 mark

d) Name any two pharmacological effects of smoking and the effects on various drugs. 2 marks

e) A 53-year-old male presents to the preoperative assessment clinic for an elective cholecystectomy. Although he presented for cardiac risk and these have been investigated and optimised, the preoperative assessment nurse contacts you as she is worried about the history of smoking 30 cigarettes per day for the last 33 years. As an anaesthetist, what would be your actions in this scenario? 2 marks

f) What are the risks in this patient for anaesthesia considering the association with smoking? 4 marks

g) What are the pharmacological options for smoking cessation that are licensed in the United Kingdom? 2 marks

h) Intraoperatively, this patient develops bronchospasm during his general anaesthesia; what drugs, including dosages, can be used to treat this? 3 marks

Q18 — Oxygenation and hyperoxia

a) What physiological factors determine the rate of fall in arterial oxygen saturation in an apnoeic patient (3 marks), and which patient groups are most likely to show a rapid fall (4 marks)? 7 marks

b) How may alveolar oxygenation, prior to intubation, be optimised during a rapid sequence induction (6 marks), and how can its effectiveness be measured (1 mark)? 7 marks

c) What are the possible respiratory complications of prolonged delivery of 100% oxygen? 2 marks

d) What are the four stages of pulmonary toxicity that occurs due to hyperoxia? 4 marks

Q19 — Antiplatelet medications

a) What are the indications for antiplatelet drugs in clinical practice? 4 marks

b) List the agents currently in clinical use. 3 marks

c) What is the mechanism of action of aspirin and phosphodiesterase inhibitors? 4 marks

d) What is the mechanism of action of ADP receptor blocking drugs and GP IIb/IIIa inhibitors? 4 marks

e) How may active bleeding be managed following the administration of one of these agents? 5 marks

Q20 — Fundoplication and laparoscopic effects

A 35-year-old patient is scheduled for an elective Nissen fundoplication.

a) List and briefly state the reasons for the cardiovascular effects of laparoscopy in the head-up position for a Nissen fundoplication. 7 marks

b) What are the respiratory effects of this surgery in the same patient? 4 marks

c) What ventilation strategies can be used to minimise these side effects? 4 marks

d) List any four benefits of laparoscopic surgery. 2 marks

e) List the risks of laparoscopic surgery. 3 marks

Q21 — Splenectomy

A 26-year-old patient with stage 4B Hodgkin's disease (spread to lymph nodes and other organs) requires an open splenectomy.

a) List the specific factors that are of importance in the preoperative planning for this patient. 6 marks

b) List the salient features of intraoperative management for this patient. 5 marks

c) Outline the options for providing postoperative analgesia for this patient and give a possible disadvantage of each. 4 marks

d) Which vaccinations should this patient receive and what is the optimal timing of these? 5 marks

Q22 — Scoliosis surgery

A 15-year-old adolescent girl is listed for surgery for the correction of scoliosis.

a) How would you diagnose adolescent idiopathic scoliosis? 2 marks

b) What is the incidence of scoliosis? 2 marks

c) What are the problems that would result due to scoliosis? 3 marks

d) What surgical procedures are available for scoliosis? 2 marks

e) What specific problems related to anaesthesia should be remembered for these surgeries? 2 marks

f) What are the intraoperative management strategies that could be considered for scoliosis surgeries? 6 marks

g) List the effects of anaesthetic agents on neurophysiological monitoring that are used during scoliosis surgeries. 3 marks

Q23 — Perioperative hypothermia

A 54-year-old male underwent a 4-hour laparotomy procedure and experienced a delayed recovery due to hypothermia.

a) What is inadvertent perioperative hypothermia (IPH)? 1 mark

b) Describe the physiology of thermoregulation. 3 marks

c) Describe the effect of anaesthesia on heat balance. 3 marks

d) What are the risk factors for IPH? 3 marks

e) List a few consequences of IPH. 3 marks

f) What steps would you take to prevent IPH preoperatively? 2 marks

g) List the measures that you would take in the operating theatre to prevent IPH. 3 marks

h) Name two pharmacological agents with doses that could be used if this patient has post-anaesthetic shivering in recovery. 2 marks

Q24 — Surgical fires

A 72-year-old gentleman is listed for laser debulking of an upper airway tumour; the procedure has a risk of surgical fire.

a) What are the three components of the fire triad required to form a fire? 3 marks

b) What are the sources of fire in an operating theatre environment? 2 marks

c) List the algorithm for fire prevention in the operating theatre. 3 marks

d) What safety measures would you consider if you are using a cuffed tracheal tube for a laser surgery in the above patient? 2 marks

e) List the types of lasers used and the tracheal tubes that could be used. 2 mark

f) What actions would you take in the unfortunate event of a surgical fire in the airway in this patient? 3 mark

g) List the actions you would take if the fire occurs outside the airway. 3 mark

h) How can we improve the culture of fire safety in operating theatres? 2 marks

Q25 — Sedation

You are asked to sedate a frightened adult patient for the insertion of dental implants.

a) Complete the table with the different levels of sedation from the American Society of Anesthesiologists' (ASA) continuum of sedation (top row) and the clinical features seen at each level (rows below). 8 marks

Table 9.1

	Minimal sedation/ anxiolysis	**Moderate sedation/ analgesia ('conscious sedation')**	**Deep sedation/ analgesia**
Responsiveness			
Airway			
Spontaneous ventilation			
Cardiovascular function			

b) Outline the drugs that may be used and their methods of administration, when providing sedation for this patient. 4 marks

c) What are the best practice principles for providing safe sedation in this patient? 8 marks

Q26 — MRI scans

You are asked to transfer an intubated intensive care patient for a magnetic resonance imaging (MRI) scan.

a) What is meant by the terms "MR safe" and "MR conditional" in relation to equipment used in the MRI scanner room? 2 marks

b) What precautions should be taken to prevent burns caused by monitoring equipment used in an MRI scanner? 4 marks

c) Describe other precautions that you should take while this patient is having an MRI scan. 8 marks

d) List any six relative/absolute contraindications to an MRI scan for any patient. 6 marks

Q27 — Pulmonary hypertension

a) Define pulmonary hypertension. 2 marks

b) List four causes of pulmonary hypertension. 2 marks

c) What are the symptoms and signs in patients with pulmonary hypertension? 3 marks

d) What are the specific anaesthetic goals when anaesthetising a patient with pulmonary hypertension? 7 marks

e) List the pharmacological treatments available for this condition. 6 marks

Q28 — Statistics, reviews and meta-analysis

A recent meta-analysis of Mallampati scoring of the airway found that it had a sensitivity of 60% and a specificity of 70%.

a) Briefly define the terms "systematic review" and "meta-analysis". 4 marks

b) Explain what is meant by sensitivity and specificity. 4 marks

c) According to this meta-analysis what is the positive predictive value of Mallampati scoring of the airway and how is it calculated? 2 marks

d) What is the possible bias with a meta-analysis? 2 marks

e) List the key steps in designing a clinical trial. 8 marks

Q29 — End-stage renal failure

a) List three of the commonest causes of end-stage renal failure (ESRF) in the United Kingdom. 3 marks

b) What complications of ESRF are of importance to the anaesthetist? 6 marks

c) What acute physiological disturbances may be seen in a patient who has just had haemodialysis? 3 marks

d) What are the key practical considerations when providing general anaesthesia for a patient with ESRF on haemodialysis? 8 marks

Q30 — Malignant hyperthermia

A healthy 39-year-old male is anaesthetised with a general anaesthetic for a laparoscopic cholecystectomy. As soon as the skin incision is made, it is noted that the core temperature is rising quickly. This is associated with a rise in $etCO_2$ and an increase in heart rate.

a) What are the differential diagnoses in this condition? 4 marks

b) What is malignant hyperthermia? 1 mark

c) Name some triggers for malignant hyperthermia. 2 marks

d) What is the pathophysiology of malignant hyperthermia? 3 marks

e) How would you manage malignant hyperthermia? 8 marks

f) How would you confirm the diagnosis of malignant hyperpyrexia? 2 marks

Q31 — Rheumatoid arthritis

A 72-year-old patient with longstanding severe rheumatoid arthritis (RhA) presents for a total knee replacement.

a) Which joints may be affected in RhA? Indicate why this is relevant to anaesthesia care. 4 marks

b) What are the effects of RhA on the following systems? 3 marks

Cardiovascular system: ______________________________

Respiratory system: ______________________________

Haematological system: ______________________________

c) List the hepatorenal, neurological and ocular manifestations of RhA. 3 marks

d) List the classes of drugs used to treat RhA. 3 marks

e) List two systemic side effects of any three medications that you listed above. 3 marks

f) Outline the preoperative investigations that are specifically indicated in this patient and the derangements that each may show. 4 marks

Q32 — Point-of-care gastric ultrasound

a) What is the incidence of pulmonary aspiration of gastric contents in elective general anaesthesia? 1 mark

b) What is the single most commonly used measure to mitigate the risk of pulmonary aspiration? 1 mark

c) Describe a few rarely used invasive methods to assess gastric contents and emptying. 3 marks

d) How can point-of-care gastric ultrasound be used in the assessment of risk for pulmonary aspiration? 2 marks

e) Describe the framework used in the performance of point-of-care gastric ultrasound. **4 marks**

f) How would you stratify the risk with the findings of a gastric ultrasound? **3 marks**

g) List a few conditions where gastric ultrasound might be difficult and explain the reasons. **3 marks**

h) What are the advantages of gastric ultrasound? **3 marks**

Chapter 10

Optional topics
QUESTIONS

Q1 — Radical nephrectomy

A 59-year-old gentleman is listed for a radical nephrectomy in the urology theatre.

a) How does a radical procedure differ from a simple nephrectomy? 2 marks

b) This gentleman has a diagnosis of renal cell carcinoma; what are the genetic or environmental risk factors for renal cell carcinoma? 2 marks

c) This patient has a history of high blood pressure, controlled on ramipril and atenolol. How would you assess him preoperatively and what considerations would be taken into account in the preoperative clinic? 4 marks

d) What are the plans that you would make for the intraoperative management of this gentleman coming in for a radical nephrectomy? 6 marks

e) What are the complications after a radical nephrectomy? 4 mark

f) What are the postoperative concerns in this patient? 2 mark

Q2 — Burns

A 45-year-old man suffered from a flame burn to his body at his work place.

a) Besides the rule of nine method, suggest two other methods for estimating the total body surface area of burn injury. 2 mark

b) Clinically, how would you differentiate a partial skin thickness burn (second degree) and full skin thickness burn (third degree)? Please give two clinical signs to contrast the difference. 4 mark

c) Name five clinical signs that may raise your suspicion of an airway burn injury. 5 mark

d) Name four factors that would affect the amount of fluid resuscitation you offer to a severely burned patient. 4 mark

e) Apart from total body surface area and depth, what other types of injury would you consider managing in a hospital with a burn facility? Please suggest two conditions. 5 mark

Q3 — Thoracoabdominal aneurysms

A 47-year-old male presents to the accident and emergency department and has a provisional diagnosis of a thoracic aortic dissection. He is haemodynamically unstable.

a) What are the differences between a true aneurysm, pseudoaneurysm and a dissection? 3 marks

b) What are the indications for elective surgery for a thoracoabdominal aortic aneurysm? 3 marks

c) How can you classify thoracoabdominal aneurysms? 2 marks

d) How can you classify aortic dissection? 4 marks

e) How would you manage the anaesthetic care for this patient? 8 marks

Q4 — Free flaps in breast surgery

A 35-year-old woman is listed for a mastectomy and free-flap breast reconstruction for breast cancer.

a) What is the difference between a radical mastectomy and breast-conserving treatment? 2 marks

b) How does sentinel lymph node biopsy differ from axillary lymph node dissection? What are the specific risks of sentinel biopsy? 4 marks

c) What are the different types of flap used for reconstruction after breast tumour excision? 4 marks

d) What are the causes of flap failure and what physiological goals are important for a healthy free flap outcome? 5 marks

e) What are the important anaesthetic considerations for this type of surgery? 5 marks

Q5 — Endovascular aneurysm repair

A 79-year-old man with a 6cm infrarenal abdominal aortic aneurysm is to undergo an endovascular aneurysm repair (EVAR). He is known to have chronic obstructive pulmonary disease.

a) What are the advantages of an EVAR compared with an open repair of the aneurysm for this patient? 6 mark

b) Which is the most important modifiable risk factor for the formation, progression and rupture of an abdominal aortic aneurysm (AAA)? 1 mark

c) What are the strongest predictors for rupture of an AAA? 2 mark

d) List the risk factors for acute kidney injury (AKI) during any EVAR procedure. 5 mark

e) Enumerate the perioperative measures to prevent AKI following EVAR. 4 mark

f) What percentage of patients develop post-implantation syndrome and what is it comprised of? 2 mark

Q6 — Orthognathic surgeries

A 24-year-old lady is listed for a bimaxillary osteotomy.

a) What are the indications for orthognathic surgery? 2 mark

b) Name any three other types of orthognathic surgeries. 3 mark

c) What would be your perioperative airway concerns with such a patient? 6 marks

d) How can blood loss be minimised in this case? 3 marks

e) What are the clinical advantages in using remifentanil for this operation? 2 marks

f) What precautions would you take to reduce the risk of a retained throat pack post-surgery? 4 marks

Q7 — Perioperative dental damage

a) List any six anaesthetic factors that predispose to perioperative dental damage. 6 marks

b) Name any four dental factors that predispose to perioperative dental damage. 4 marks

c) You have anaesthetised a 22-year-old man and you notice a missing front tooth after intubation. What would be your initial management of this situation? 6 marks

d) How would you follow this patient up? 4 marks

Q8 — Perioperative medicine and prehabilitation

A 68-year-old male presents to the preoperative assessment clinic for a radical prostatectomy. He is a known hypertensive on ramipril 10mg, bisoprolol 2.5mg and a GTN spray as required. He complains of shortness of breath and, rarely, palpitations on moderate exercise as per his history. He smokes 10 cigarettes per day. His Body Mass Index is 42.3kg/m^2. He has a sedentary lifestyle and drinks five units of alcohol per week. Due to his executive job, his activities are restricted.

a) What is the role of perioperative medicine in this person presenting for a major surgery? 2 marks

b) What is the role of cardiopulmonary exercise testing (CPET) in this individual and what data does it provide? 2 marks

c) What simple bedside tests can you do for this purpose before the CPET in the assessment clinic? 2 marks

d) Name any two risk stratification tools used for surgical outcomes. 2 marks

e) If there is adequate time to prepare in the patient described above, what techniques of prehabilitation can you use? 4 marks

f) What other comorbidities could be managed in the prehabilitation clinic? 2 marks

g) What fluid management technique would you use intraoperatively in the operating theatre? 2 marks

h) What concerns would you have in the postoperative period for this patient and what techniques would you use for optimal recovery? 4 marks

Q9 — Carotid endarterectomy

A 56-year-old man is listed for a carotid endarterectomy 10 days after suffering a cerebrovascular accident.

a) What are the advantages of performing this procedure under regional anaesthesia? 4 marks

b) What are the disadvantages of using regional anaesthesia for this procedure? 4 marks

c) What local or regional anaesthetic techniques may be used? 3 marks

d) How can the patient's risk of perioperative cerebrovascular accident be minimised? 6 marks

e) Following this procedure, what other specific postoperative complications may occur? 3 marks

Q10 — Renal transplant

A patient is scheduled to receive a cadaveric renal transplant.

a) What would be the salient features for preoperative investigation and optimisation of this patient, specific to chronic kidney disease? 8 marks

b) Intraoperatively, how could you optimise the function of the transplanted kidney? 6 marks

c) List three options to manage this patient's postoperative pain. 3 marks

d) List the common postoperative analgesic drugs to be avoided or used with caution. 3 marks

Q11 — Head and neck cancer and free flap transfer

A 54-year-old patient with a base of tongue cancer presents for a hemiglossectomy and radial forearm free flap reconstruction.

a) List any four aetiological factors implicated in head and neck cancers. 2 marks

b) Which specific factors must the anaesthetist consider when assessing this patient prior to surgery? 3 marks

c) What are the preoperative airway considerations? 3 marks

d) What are the causes of impaired nutrition in these patients? 2 marks

e) How is the nutritional status optimised in the perioperative period? 1 mark

f) What scoring system is recommended to predict cardiac risk in the perioperative period? What is the risk associated with head and neck surgeries? 2 marks

g) List the benefits of a free flap reconstruction. 2 marks

h) What are the absolute contraindications for a free flap transfer and why? 2 marks

i) What are the intraoperative anaesthetic considerations? 3 marks

Q12 — Direct oral anticoagulants

A 71-year-old male is scheduled for an elective abdominal aneurysm repair. Thoracic epidural analgesia is planned perioperatively. The patient is on rivaroxaban and aspirin.

a) What are the oral anticoagulants that you are aware of? 1 mark

b) What are the advantages and disadvantages of warfarin as compared with direct oral anticoagulants (DOACs)? 2 marks

c) Name a few indications for DOACs. 2 marks

d) List the mechanism of action of oral anticoagulants. 2 marks

e) How long should you withhold oral anticoagulants perioperatively? 2 marks

f) When would you stop a DOAC before neuraxial anaesthesia? 2 marks

g) When would you consider warfarin bridging and how would you organise this in a patient who takes warfarin? 2 marks

h) How would you bridge a DOAC? 2 marks

i) Which group of patients would you consider as high risk for perioperative thrombotic risk? 1 mark

j) What tests would you use to test the efficacy of an anticoagulant? 2 marks

k) How would you reverse the action of an oral anticoagulant? 2 marks

Q13 — Regional anaesthesia for the eye

a) List the nerves supplying the orbit. 2 marks

b) What are the contraindications to regional anaesthesia for the eye? 5 marks

c) What is the dose and mechanism of action of hyaluronidase, added to the local anaesthetic mix for eye blocks? 2 marks

d) Describe the guidance on the use of anticoagulants and antiplatelet medications in patients scheduled for eye surgery. 5 marks

e) List any six NICE recommendations (on the day of surgery) to prevent wrong lens implants. 6 marks

Q14 — Penetrating eye injury and regional block

A healthy 32-year-old male with an ASA I physical status score was involved in a road traffic accident and suffered a penetrating eye injury.

a) What factors determine the intraocular pressure in a healthy eye? 5 marks

b) What key points would you need to know when assessing this patient preoperatively? 3 marks

c) The patient requires urgent surgery. Discuss your specific intraoperative management. 4 marks

d) What are the contraindications to perform a regional block in an elective ophthalmic surgery? 5 marks

e) What different types of regional block are suitable for ophthalmic surgery? 3 marks

Q15 — Robotic surgeries

a) What are the preoperative considerations for a patient who is listed for robotic surgery? 3 marks

b) What are the main physiological considerations in robotic surgery procedures? 3 marks

c) What are the main anaesthetic considerations for robotic surgery? 8 marks

d) What are the possible risks and complications associated with robotic surgery? 4 marks

e) List four specialty surgeries that could be done with robotic surgery. 2 marks

Section 2
Answers

Chapter 11

Neuroanaesthesia

ANSWERS

Q1 — Cerebrospinal fluid physiology

a) Describe the production and circulation of cerebrospinal fluid (CSF). 3 marks

CSF is produced by the choroid plexus in the lateral, third and fourth ventricles by:

- Plasma filtration through capillary fenestrations.
- Active transport across the blood/CSF barrier.

CSF circulates through the following structures:

- Lateral ventricles.
- Foramen of Monro.
- Third ventricle.
- Aqueduct of Sylvius.
- Fourth ventricle.
- Foramina of Magendie and Luschka.
- Cisterna magna.
- Spinal and cerebral subarachnoid space.

CSF is absorbed by arachnoid granulations into cerebral venous sinuses.

b) How does the intracranial pressure affect the production and absorption of CSF? 2 marks

Compensatory mechanisms with a rise in ICP include:

- Spatial compensation — displacement of CSF from the cranial into the spinal subarachnoid space.
- Increased absorption of CSF.
- Does not affect the production of CSF.

c) Give five differentiating features of CSF vs. plasma with regards to its biochemistry. 5 marks

Table 11.1

	Plasma	**CSF**
Glucose	3-5mmol/L	2.4-4.5mmol/L
Sodium	135-145mmol/L	144-152mmol/L
Potassium	3.5-5mmol/L	2-3mmol/L
Chloride	95-105mmol/L	123-128mmol/L
Calcium	2.2-2.6mmol/L	1.1-1.3mmol/L
Bicarbonate	24-28mmol/L	24-28mmol/L
Urea	2.5-6.5mmol/L	2-7mmol/L
Protein	45-60g/L	0.3g/L
Osmolality	280-310mosm/L	280-310mosm/L
pH	7.4	7.3

d) List any four indications for lumbar puncture. 4 marks

Diagnostic indications:

- Diagnosis of meningitis.
- Suspected CNS infections, e.g. encephalitis.
- Suspected subarachnoid haemorrhage with a negative CT.
- Normal pressure hydrocephalus.
- Idiopathic intracranial hypertension.
- Injection of contrast media for myelography and cisternography.

Therapeutic indications:

- Subarachnoid block.
- Intrathecal chemotherapy.
- Intrathecal antibiotics.

e) Name any six factors that predispose to the development of a postdural puncture headache after lumbar puncture. 6 marks

Patient factors:

- Young age.
- Female.
- Pregnancy.

Equipment factors:

- Large diameter needles.
- Cutting needles that transect the dural fibres.

Operator factors:

- Multiple attempts.
- Perpendicular orientation of the bevel of a spinal or epidural needle leads to a reduction in the incidence of postdural puncture headache.
- Intermittent technique for epidural insertion.
- Identifying loss of resistance with air rather than saline.

References

1. Krovvidi H, Flint G, Williams AV. Perioperative management of hydrocephalus. *Br J Anaesth Education* 2018; 18(5): 140-6.
2. Tameem A, Krovvidi H. Cerebral physiology. *Br J Anaesth CEACCP* 2013; 13(4): 113-8.
3. Turnbull DK, Shepherd DB. Post-dural puncture headache: pathogenesis, prevention and treatment. *Br J Anaesth* 2003; 91(5): 718-29.
4. Smith T, Pinnock C, Lin T, Jones R, Eds. *Fundamentals of Anaesthesia*, 3rd ed. Cambridge: Cambridge University Press, 2009.
5. Warrell W, Cox TM, Firth JD, Eds. *Oxford Textbook of Medicine*, 5th ed. Oxford: Oxford University Press, 2010.

Q2 — Brainstem death and organ donation

A 20-year-old patient in a neurointensive care unit satisfies the criteria for brainstem death and has been accepted as an organ donor.

a) List the main adverse cardiovascular changes associated with brainstem death. 5 marks

- An initial increase in arterial BP to maintain CPP.
- Effect of pontine ischaemia and a hyperadrenergic response:
  - hypertension and bradycardia (as part of Cushing's triad with irregular respiration);
  - an increase in right and left ventricular afterload.
- Effect of foramen magnum herniation and loss of spinal sympathetic activity:
  - vasodilation;
  - reduced cardiac output;
  - reduced afterload and preload decreasing aortic diastolic pressure.
- Effect of pituitary ischaemia:
  - diabetes insipidus — hypovolaemia and electrolyte imbalance.
- Arrhythmias due to electrolyte imbalance, acidosis and catecholamines.

b) What are the physiological goals (with values) required to ensure optimisation of this donor? 7 marks

CVS targets:

- Heart rate 60-120 beats/min.
- Systolic arterial pressure >100mmHg.
- Mean arterial pressure >70mmHg but <95mmHg.
- Central venous pressure 6-10mmHg.
- Pulmonary artery occlusion pressure 10-15mmHg.
- Stroke volume variation <10%.

- Cardiac index >2.1L/min/m^2.
- Mixed venous saturation >60%.

Mechanical ventilation targets:

- Tidal volume: 6-8ml/kg.
- PEEP >5cm H_2O.
- Peak inspiratory pressure <25cm H_2O.
- pH 7.35-7.45.
- PaO_2 >10kPa.
- $PaCO_2$ 4.5-6.0kPa.
- SpO_2 >95% for the lowest FiO_2, ideally <0.4.

Renal management:

- Avoid hypovolaemia and nephrotoxic drugs.
- Adequate renal perfusion pressure.

Hepatic management:

- Restore hepatic glycogen stores — continue enteral feeding.
- Serum sodium <155mmol/L.
- Avoid a high PEEP to reduce hepatic congestion.
- Central venous pressure 6-10mmHg.

Miscellaneous:

- Temperature >34°C.
- Serum glucose 4.0-8.0mmol/L.
- Correct coagulopathies.

c) Outline the measures that may be used to achieve the needed goals. 5 marks

Cardiovascular management:

- TTE or continuous cardiac output monitoring.
- Esmolol, GTN, and SNP to manage hypertension.
- Intravenous fluids and vasopressin to manage hypotension.
- Amiodarone for tachyarrhythmias.
- Bradyarrhythmias are treated with adrenaline or isoprenaline.
- Thyroid hormone replacement to improve cardiac function.

Respiratory management:

- Lung protective ventilation strategies.
- 30° head-up tilt, regular tracheal suction, regular rotation.
- Avoid a positive fluid balance.
- Methylprednisolone to minimise extravascular lung water.
- Bronchoscopy for directed suction.
- CXR to detect neurogenic pulmonary oedema.

Renal management:

- Avoid hypovolaemia and nephrotoxic drugs.

Hepatic management:

- Restoring liver glycogen with adequate nutrition.
- Serum sodium <155mmol/L to avoid osmosis from recipient to donor cells.
- Avoid a high PEEP to reduce hepatic congestion.
- Central venous pressure 6-10mmHg.

d) Name any three medications that you might use to optimise the endocrine system. 3 marks

- Methylprednisolone.
- Thyroid hormone T3.
- Vasopressin.
- Desmopressin to treat DI.
- Insulin infusion.

References

1. Gordon JK, McKinlay J. Physiological changes after brain stem death and management of the heart-beating donor. *Br J Anaesth CEACCP* 2012; 12(5): 225-9.

Q3 — Status epilepticus

You are asked to review a 27-year-old male who is a known epileptic in convulsive status epilepticus.

a) Name two opioids contraindicated in seizures. 2 marks

- Alfentanil — enhances EEG activity.
- Pethidine/meperidine — metabolite nor-meperidine is a pro-convulsant.
- Tramadol — lowers the seizure threshold.

b) What are the implications of neuromuscular blocking drugs in epileptic patients? 2 marks

- Succinylcholine — in prolonged status epilepticus, it can cause dangerous hyperkalaemia.
- Non-depolarising NMBAs — enzyme-inducing effects of antiepileptic drugs (AEDs) may cause resistance to the effects of aminosteroid neuromuscular blockers, such as rocuronium, pancuronium, and vecuronium.
- Laudanosine, a metabolite of atracurium, has epileptogenic potential.

c) Define convulsive status epilepticus. 1 mark

Status epilepticus is defined as continuous seizure activity of at least 30 minutes' duration or intermittent seizure activity of at least 30 minutes' duration during which consciousness is not regained.

d) What drugs, including doses, are used during the various stages of status epilepticus? 5 marks

Premonitory stage (prehospital or <5 minutes):

- Diazepam 10-15mg PR, repeat after 15 minutes. OR
- Midazolam 10mg buccal.

Early stage (5-10 minutes):

- Lorazepam 0.1mg/kg, repeat after 10-20 minutes.
- Give the usual antiepileptic drugs.
- Glucose 50ml 50% IV and thiamine 250mg IV if there is suspected alcohol abuse or malnutrition.

Established stage (0-60 minutes):

- Phenytoin IV 15-18mg/kg at 50mg/min.

e) What investigations would you consider in a patient with status epilepticus? 2 mark

- Blood investigations — arterial blood gases and venous blood sampling for glucose, calcium, and magnesium levels; renal and liver function; a full blood count; clotting screen; AED level assay; and toxicology screen.
- Brain imaging — CT, MRI.
- Microbiology.
- Lumbar puncture.
- EEG.

f) Sixty minutes after your initial management, the patient continues to be in status epilepticus. What would be your further management? 5 mark

- General anaesthesia, intubation and ventilation with:
  - propofol (1-2mg/kg bolus, followed by an infusion); OR
  - thiopentone (3-5mg/kg bolus, followed by an infusion); OR
  - midazolam (0.1-0.2mg/kg bolus, followed by an infusion).
- Intensive care management.
- EEG monitoring.
- Intracranial pressure monitoring where appropriate.

- CNS imaging and LP where appropriate.
- Initiate long-term, maintenance antiepileptic drugs.
- Anaesthetic continued for 12-24 hours after the last clinical or EEG seizures and gradually weaned.

g) What are the complications associated with refractory convulsive status epilepticus? 3 marks

- Excitotoxic CNS injury.
- Hyperthermia.
- Pulmonary oedema.
- Arrhythmias.
- Cardiovascular collapse.
- Acute kidney and liver injury.
- Rhabdomyolysis.
- Fractures.

References

1. Carter EL, Adapa RM. Adult epilepsy and anaesthesia. *Br J Anaesth Education* 2015; 15(3): 111-7.
2. Epilepsies: diagnosis and management. NICE clinical guideline, CG137. London: National Institute for Health and Care Excellence, 2018. https://www.nice.org.uk/guidance/cg137. Accessed on 25th June 2019.

Q4 — Delirium in critical care

a) Define delirium. 2 mark

Delirium is defined as a disturbance of consciousness and a change in cognition that develops over a short period of time.

b) List the key clinical features that are used to diagnose delirium in critical care. 4 mark

- Inattentiveness — difficulty following instructions or easily distracted.
- Disorientation — to time, place or person.
- Hallucinations and delusions.
- Psychosis.
- Psychomotor agitation or retardation — agitation requiring the use of drugs or restraints.
- Inappropriate speech or mood.
- Sleep/wake cycle disturbance.
- Symptom fluctuation.

c) List any six risk factors for delirium in an intensive care patient. 3 mark

Patient characteristics:

- Increasing age.
- Visual or hearing impairment.

Pre-existing cognition:

- Depression.
- Dementia.
- History of delirium.

Functional impairment:

- Poor oral intake of diet and fluid.
- Immobility.
- A history of falls.

Drugs:

- Alcohol and other substance withdrawal.
- Narcotics, including tramadol and meperidine.
- Drugs with anticholinergic effects.
- Steroids, digoxin and diuretics.

Medical conditions:

- Electrolyte disturbance, including hypomagnesaemia.
- Chronic renal and liver failure.
- Neurological disease, including stroke.
- Trauma.

d) List some methods of diagnosis and assessment of delirium. 1 mark

- Confusion Assessment Method for the Intensive Care Unit (CAM-ICU).
- Intensive Care Delirium Screening Checklist (ICDSC).
- Diagnosis by a psychiatrist using DSM IV.

e) In a delirious critical care patient, what are the most common environmental factors that are potentially treatable? 3 marks

- Correct visual and hearing impairment with glasses and hearing aids.
- Orientate the patient regularly.
- Promote sleep hygiene.
- Mobilise.
- Use physical restraints only to prevent harm.

f) What medical factors would you correct to treat/prevent delirium? 3 marks

- Avoid hypoxia.
- Correct metabolic problems (dehydration, acidosis, electrolyte disturbances).
- Treat any infection.
- Administer adequate analgesia.
- Remove lines if not needed.
- Sedation hold and trial of breathing if intubated and ventilated.

g) When is pharmacological treatment indicated and which classes of drugs can be used? 4 marks

Pharmacological treatment is indicated when:

- The person is distressed.
- Poses a risk to themselves or others.
- Verbal and non-verbal de-escalation techniques are ineffective or inappropriate.

The classes of drugs used are:

- D2 receptor antagonist — haloperidol.
- Atypical antipsychotics — olanzapine, quetiapine.
- Avoid benzodiazepines except in delirium due to alcohol withdrawal — lorazepam.

References

1. Delirium: prevention, diagnosis and management. NICE clinical guideline, CG103. London: National Institute for Health and Care Excellence, 2010. https://www.nice.org.uk/guidance/cg103. Accessed on 25th June 2019.

2. King J, Gratrix A. Delirium in intensive care. *Br J Anaesth CEACCP* 2009; 9(5): 144-7.
3. Lloyd DG, Ma D, Vizcaychipi MP. Cognitive decline after anaesthesia and critical care. *Br J Anaesth CEACCP* 2012; 12(3): 105-9.

Q5 — Near-drowning

A 20-year-old man is brought to the emergency department having been pulled from a river following a near-drowning.

a) What are the effects of near-drowning on the respiratory and cardiovascular systems? 2 marks

Respiratory system:

- Wash out of surfactant causes atelectasis and lung collapse.
- Osmotic gradients cause alveolar and interstitial oedema.
- Bronchospasm.
- Acute emphysema due to alveolar rupture.
- Toxins in water cause alveolar injury.
- ALI and ARDS.

Cardiovascular system:

- Hypoxia and hypothermia trigger catecholamine release.
- Catecholamines cause vasoconstriction and acidosis.
- Hypothermia causes arrhythmias and cardiac failure.

b) What are the effects on other systems? 1 mark

- CNS — hypoxia and cerebral oedema.
- Haematology — lactic acidosis, haemolysis, DIC.
- Renal — AKI due to myoglobinuria, lactic acidosis, hypoperfusion.

c) List the relevant features in the history that you would elicit in this patient. 3 marks

Victim information:

- Precipitating events — arrhythmia, myocardial infarction, seizure, non-accidental injury, etc.
- Intoxication — alcohol, drugs.
- Vomiting.

Scene information:

- Mechanism of injury, submersion time, water type, temperature, contaminants.

Pre-hospital care:

- Initial ABC and GCS, CPR — time started, any delay, time to return of spontaneous respiration and circulation.

d) List the investigations that you would perform in this particular patient. 3 marks

- Bloods — ABG, electrolytes, renal function, glucose, FBC, LFTs, coagulation screen, CK, osmolarity, alcohol level, toxic screen.
- ECG — rate, rhythm, evidence of ischaemia, J waves of hypothermia.
- Radiology — CXR, C-spine imaging, CT head, trauma imaging.
- Microbiology — sputum/tracheal aspirates, blood culture.

e) How would you treat hypothermia in this patient? 4 marks

Mild hypothermia (32-35°C) — passive rewarming:

- Remove wet clothing, apply an insulating cover.

Moderate hypothermia (30-32°C) and severe hypothermia (<30°C) — active rewarming:

- Active external rewarming — warmed pads, forced air warming blanket, radiant heater.
- Active internal warming — humidified warm inspired gases, warmed IV fluids, body cavity lavage, extracorporeal methods such as haemodialysis and cardiopulmonary bypass.

When return of cardiac output is achieved, in comatose patients, rewarming to 32-34°C is recommended.

f) What are the considerations for ventilatory strategies for this patient? 4 marks

- Lung protective ventilation strategies:
  - tidal volume of 6ml/kg,
  - plateau pressure below 30cm H_2O;
  - PEEP and FIO_2 titrated to PaO_2;
  - permissive hypercapnia may interfere with neuroprotection.
- Consider the use of ECMO/surfactant therapy/nitric oxide/prostacyclin in ARDS.
- Prophylactic antibiotics if submerged in grossly contaminated water.

g) Outline your neuroprotective strategies for this patient. 3 marks

- Comatose patients should be rewarmed to 32-34°C and this mild hypothermia maintained for 12-24 hours.
- Prevent secondary brain injury:
  - 30° head-up tilt;
  - avoid hypoxia, maintain normocapnia;
  - maintain adequate MAP;
  - glucose control (target of 5-10mmol/L);
  - prompt treatment of seizures.

References

1. Carter E, Sinclair R. Drowning. *Br J Anaesth CEACCP* 2011; 11(6): 210-3.

Q6 — Acromegaly and hypophysectomy

A 54-year-old male with acromegaly presents for a transsphenoidal hypophysectomy.

a) What is acromegaly? 1 mark

Acromegaly is a chronic, progressive, multisystem disease caused by an excess of growth hormone (GH) after puberty.

b) List the clinical features of acromegaly which are of relevance to the anaesthetist. 3 mark

Airway:

- Soft tissue proliferation in the upper airway — airway obstruction.
- OSA.
- Subglottic narrowing.

Respiratory system:

- Kyphoscoliosis.
- Proximal myopathy.

Cardiovascular system:

- Refractory hypertension.
- LVH and IHD.
- Arrhythmias and heart block.
- Cardiomyopathy and biventricular dysfunction.

c) What are the endocrine manifestations of pituitary adenomas? 1 mark

- Pituitary adenomas secrete prolactin, ACTH, TSH, causing hyperpituitarism.
- Compress normal tissue and loss of other hormones, ACTH, TSH, ADH, causing hypopituitarism.
- DM.

d) What other clinical presentations of a pituitary adenoma may be encountered? 2 marks

- Headache.
- Bitemporal hemianopia.
- Hydrocephalus.
- Hypopituitarism/hyperpituitarism.

e) What are the specific preoperative considerations for anaesthetising this patient? 4 marks

- Anticipate and prepare for a difficult airway.
- Assess and optimise the cardiorespiratory system.
- Endocrine review to assess pituitary dysfunction.
- CT of the head to exclude hydrocephalus.
- Visual field defects are documented.
- Continue hormonal and antihypertensive therapy.
- Warn about postoperative nasal obstruction due to nasal packs.

f) What are your considerations during induction of anaesthesia for this patient? 2 marks

- Airway adjuncts including AFOI to manage a difficult airway.
- Difficult IV access, due to soft tissue proliferation in peripheries.
- A smaller sized armoured ETT (in view of subglottic narrowing).

- A throat pack is inserted.
- Vasoconstrictor nasal drops to improve surgical access.

g) What are your concerns during maintenance of anaesthesia and emergence? 3 marks

Maintenance:

- Sitting position — if a transsphenoidal approach is used.
- Risk of venous air embolism.
- Remifentanil infusion for analgesia.
- Neuromuscular monitoring and complete paralysis.
- Padding pressure points.
- The use of lumbar drains to inject saline and facilitate the descent of the pituitary gland.
- Damage to the carotid artery or cavernous sinus.
- Antiemetics.

Emergence:

- Clear blood and CSF from the airway.
- Avoid coughing during extubation.

h) What are the postoperative considerations after a transsphenoidal hypophysectomy? 2 marks

- Monitored in the high dependency unit.
- Monitor GCS and visual field defects — radiological investigations/surgical exploration if deterioration occurs.
- CPAP for OSA is contraindicated as it causes tension pneumocephalus.
- Transient DI.
- SIADH.
- Steroid and other hormonal replacement therapy.

i) What are the advantages and disadvantages of a transsphenoidal hypophysectomy approach? 2 marks

Advantages:

- Minimal surgical trauma and blood loss.
- Direct access to the gland.
- Avoidance of the generic hazards of a craniotomy.

Complications:

- Persistent CSF rhinorrhoea and the associated risk of postoperative meningitis.
- Transient DI.
- Panhypopituitarism.
- Vascular damage.
- Cranial nerve injury.
- Cerebral ischaemia.
- Stroke.

References

1. Menon R, Murphy PG, Lindley AM. Anaesthesia and pituitary disease. *Br J Anaesth CEACCP* 2011; 11(4): 133-7.

Q7 — Intracranial pressure physiology

a) What is a normal intracranial pressure (ICP)? 2 mark

5-15mmHg in the supine position.

b) Describe a normal ICP waveform. 3 mark

A normal ICP waveform is pulsatile, reflecting respiratory and cardiac cycles.

The cardiac component has three peaks: P1, P2 and P3:

- P1 (percussion wave) — correlating with arterial pulsation.
- P2 (tidal wave) — generated by arterial pulsation and resistance from intracranial parenchyma.
- P3 (dicrotic wave) — reflects closure of the aortic valve.

The respiratory component is generated by changes in intrathoracic pressure caused by respiration.

c) How does the waveform change with increased ICP? 3 mark

As intracranial compliance decreases, the following pathological waves appear:

- A wave — plateau-shaped, suggesting low brain compliance, amplitude 50-100mmHg, lasting 5-20 minutes.
- B waves — rhythmic oscillations, seen in patients on mechanical ventilation, suggesting low brain compliance, amplitude <50mmHg, occur every 1-2 minutes.
- C waves — non-pathological, rhythmic oscillations, synchronous with variations in arterial pressure, amplitude <20mmHg, occur every 4-8 minutes.

d) What are the anatomical compensatory changes to a raised ICP? 4 marks

- The intracranial contents can be divided into three compartments: brain volume 85%, cerebrospinal fluid volume 10%, and blood 5%.
- The Monroe-Kelly hypothesis states that an increase in volume of one of the compartments is compensated by a decrease in volume of the other two.
- Compensatory mechanisms include:
  - a decrease in cerebral blood volume;
  - movement of CSF from the cranial to the spinal subarachnoid space;
  - increased absorption of CSF.

e) What are the symptoms and signs of a raised ICP? 4 marks

Symptoms:

- Headache.
- Vomiting.
- Focal neurology.
- Seizures.
- Agitation.
- Drowsiness.
- Coma.

Signs:

- Papilloedema.
- Pupillary dilatation.
- Increasing BP.
- Bradycardia.
- Cheyne-Stokes breathing.
- Decorticate then decerebrate posturing.

f) List the methods to monitor ICP in the intensive care unit. 4 mark

- Intraventricular catheter (gold standard).
- Intraparenchymal catheters.
- Subdural pressure transducers.
- Extradural transducers.

References

1. Tameem A, Krovvidi H. Cerebral physiology. *Br J Anaesth CEACCP* 2013; 13(4): 113-8.
2. Elwishi M, Dinsmore J. Monitoring the brain. *Br J Anaesth CEACCP* 2019; 19(2): 54-9.
3. Pattinson K, Wynne-Jones G, Imray CHE. Monitoring intracranial pressure, perfusion and metabolism. *Br J Anaesth CEACCP* 2005; 5(4): 130-3.
4. Allman K, Wilson I, O'Donnell A, Eds. *Oxford Handbook of Anaesthesia*, 4th ed. Oxford: Oxford University Press, 2016.

Q8 — Cerebral oxygenation and metabolism

A 59-year-old male is admitted to the neurocritical care unit with a head injury. He has an intraventricular bolt inserted for monitoring and measurement of intracranial pressure.

a) What are the advantages and disadvantages of measuring ICP using an intraventricular catheter? 4 marks

Advantages:

- Provides global measurement of ICP.
- Allows therapeutic drainage of CSF.
- Allows for the administration of intrathecal drugs.

Disadvantages:

- Infection.
- A difficulty placing the catheter in patients with small ventricles and cerebral oedema.

b) How is cerberal perfusion pressure (CPP) calculated? What is the optimal value recommended for favourable outcomes in intensive care? At what level must the transducers be zeroed to measure CPP? 3 marks

- CPP = MAP - (ICP or CVP).
- The optimal recommended value is 60-70mmHg.
- Arterial and intracranial pressure transducers must be zeroed at the level of the foramen of Monro or the external auditory meatus.

c) What are the methods used to measure cerebral oxygenation? What are the principles and the clinical applications? 3 marks

- Jugular venous oxygen saturation — a catheter tip is placed in the jugular venous bulb on the side of the pathology. Spectrophotometry helps continuous measurement. Used in severe traumatic brain injury (TBI) to guide intervention.
- Near infrared spectroscopy — uses the principle of the Beer-Lambert law. Used in TBI and intraoperatively for cardiac and carotid surgery.
- Using flexible microcatheters placed in the brain parenchyma — measures tissue oxygenation using a polarographic technique similar to the Clark electrode. Used in TBI.

d) What are the methods used to measure cerebral blood flow? 3 marks

- Transcranial Doppler and transcranial colour-coded duplex.
- Imaging methods:
  - CT perfusion;
  - xenon-enhanced CT;
  - perfusion-weighted MRI;
  - positive emission tomography.

e) What are the clinical applications of transcranial Doppler? 3 marks

- To monitor vasospasm after SAH.
- Detection of microemboli.
- Intraoperative monitoring during carotid artery surgery.
- Estimation of ICP.

f) How is cerebral metabolism monitored? What are the substrates measured? 4 marks

- Cerebral metabolism is measured by cerebral microdialysis. Microdialysis catheters are inserted into the brain parenchyma and substrates diffusing from the parenchyma into the catheter are measured.

- The substrates measured are:
  - energy-related metabolites — glucose, lactate, pyruvate;
  - neurotransmitters — glutamate, aspartate;
  - markers of cellular degradation — glycerol and potassium;
  - exogenous substances — drugs.

References

1. Elwishi M, Dinsmore J. Monitoring the brain. *Br J Anaesth Education* 2019; 19(2): 54-9.

Q9 — Posterior fossa tumour and air embolism

A 34-year-old man is scheduled for a posterior fossa tumour excision.

a) List four patient positions that might be employed for this operation. 2 marks

- Lateral.
- Prone.
- Supine with head turned to the opposite side.
- Sitting.
- Park bench.

b) List five potential intraoperative and two postoperative problems that are associated with a posterior fossa craniotomy. 4 marks

Intraoperative problems:

- Cardiovascular instability.
- Venous air embolism.
- Pneumocephalus.
- Macroglossia.
- Quadriplegia.

Postoperative problems:

- Lower cranial nerves palsy — risk of aspiration.
- PONV.

c) What is the mechanism of cardiovascular instability in posterior cranial fossa tumour surgery? 2 marks

- Sitting position — venous pooling of blood in the lower limbs.
- Surgical proximity to vital structures in the pons and upper medulla.

d) What are the contraindications to the sitting position? 2 marks

Absolute contraindications:

- Ventriculo-atrial shunt.
- Right to left heart shunt.

Relative contraindications:

- Patent foramen ovale.
- Uncontrolled hypertension.
- Extremes of age.
- Severe autonomic neuropathy.

e) What monitoring techniques can specifically detect the presence of venous air embolism during surgery? For each method used, give the features that would indicate the diagnosis. 6 marks

- Precordial Doppler — to detect air in the cardiac chambers by sensing changes in blood velocity and density.
- Transoesophageal ECHO and Doppler — to detect the presence of air in the cardiac chambers.
- End-tidal carbon dioxide — $etCO_2$ decreases due to an increase in dead space ventilation.
- End-tidal nitrogen — end-tidal nitrogen increases due to a release of nitrogen from the emboli into the lungs.
- Transcranial Doppler — for the detection of air emboli.
- Pulmonary artery catheters — to note an increase in pulmonary artery pressure.
- Oesophageal stethoscope — to detect a mill-wheel murmur.
- Central venous pressure — to detect an increase in central venous pressure.
- Pulse oximeter — to detect a decrease in oxygen saturation.

f) How would you manage a significant venous air embolism in this patient? 4 marks

Immediate resuscitation:

- ABC.

Prevent further air entrainment:

- Inform the surgeon and flood the field with saline-soaked gauze.
- The suspected air entry point should be sealed.

Remove or halt the process of air entrained:

- Stop nitrous oxide if in use, and use 100% oxygen.
- If possible, position the operative field below the level of the heart to prevent further air entrainment.
- Perform the Durant manoeuvre — a partial left lateral position to prevent air lock in the right ventricle.
- Aspirate air from the right atrium through the central venous catheter.

References

1. Jagannathan S, Krovvidi H. Anaesthetic considerations for posterior fossa surgery. *Br J Anaesth CEACCP* 2014; 14(5): 202-6.
2. Webber S, Andrzejowski J, Francis G. Gas embolism in anaesthesia. *Br J Anaesth CEACCP* 2002; 2(2): 53-7.

Q10 — Neuroradiology anaesthesia

An adult patient requires angiography and interventional radiology for a cerebral aneurysm.

a) List any six intracranial neuroradiological procedures. 3 marks

- Embolisation of cerebral arteriovenous malformations and aneurysms.
- Intracerebral chemotherapy for head and neck tumours.
- Sclerotherapy of venous angiomas.
- Balloon angioplasty, carotid artery stenting and venous stenting.
- Embolisation of intracranial tumours.
- Thrombolysis and thrombectomy after a stroke.
- Stereotactic-guided neurosurgery — deep brain stimulation for movement disorders.
- Implantation of intracranial electrodes for telemetry.
- Temporal lobe resections for epilepsy.

b) What potential problems may be encountered while anaesthetising a patient in the angiography suite? 3 marks

- Problems with remote site anaesthesia — unfamiliar environment, lack of a full range of equipment, lack of familiarity with the assistance provided or procedure undertaken, difficulties with communication and the non-availability of immediate senior assistance.
- Radiation protection for the patient and staff.
- Contrast-induced nephropathy.
- Large-volume flush — fluid overload or bladder distension.
- Anaesthetist and machine are away from the patient and the table moves frequently — long ventilator tubing and IV lines are required.
- Intra-hospital transfer between the intensive care unit and angiography suite.

c) What are the specific preoperative anaesthetic considerations? 3 marks

- History and effects of the intracranial lesion on the various systems.
- Drug allergy to iodine, shellfish, or contrast to be elicited.
- The patient should be examined for Glasgow Coma Scale score, pupil size and reactivity, and focal neurological deficits.
- Imaging (CT head, MRI) should be viewed.
- Renal function (urea, creatinine and electrolytes) should be tested before the administration of contrast. Metformin should be withheld post-contrast if the eGFR is <60ml/minute.
- Pregnancy test — due to a high dose of ionising radiation exposure.

d) What are the intraoperative anaesthetic considerations? 3 marks

- Large-bore intravenous access.
- Cerebral protection strategies.
- The combination of propofol and remifentanil or sevoflurane and remifentanil used.
- General anaesthesia with controlled ventilation preferred.
- Intra-arterial BP for monitoring coagulation and blood gases.
- Intravenous heparin 70-100 U/kg to maintain ACT 2-3 times the baseline.
- Temperature monitoring for long procedures in a cold angiography suite.
- A large-volume flush is used necessitating urinary catheterisation.
- Nasogastric tube for the administration of aspirin and clopidogrel.

e) Outline your management if haemorrhage occurs during the procedure. 3 marks

- Reverse heparin with protamine.
- Decrease bleeding by lowering blood pressure (to the level before the bleed).

- Control ICP with hyperventilation, head elevation, steroids and osmotic agents.
- Control seizures.
- Once the bleeding is controlled, the pressure may be raised to check for leaks.
- An external ventricular drain may be required.
- If coiling is unsuccessful, a rescue craniotomy and clipping will be required.

f) What are the effects of a subarachnoid haemorrhage on the cardiovascular and respiratory systems? What are the metabolic derangements? 5 marks

Cardiovascular system:

- Massive catecholamine release.
- Dysrhythmias.
- Abnormal ECG morphology (T inversion, ST depression, Q waves, U waves, and prolonged QT).
- Elevated cardiac enzymes.
- Left ventricular dysfunction.
- Pulmonary oedema.

Respiratory system:

- Atelectasis and pneumonia.
- Neurogenic pulmonary oedema.

Metabolic derangements:

- Syndrome of inappropriate ADH secretion.
- Dehydration.
- Hypomagnesaemia, hypernatraemia, hyponatraemia, hypokalaemia, and hypocalcaemia.

References

1. Patel S, Reddy U. Anaesthesia for interventional neuroradiology. *Br J Anaesth Education* 2016; 16(5): 147-52.
2. Dorairaj IL, Hancock SM. Anaesthesia for interventional neuroradiology. *Br J Anaesth CEACCP* 2008; 8(3): 86-9.

Chapter 12

Obstetric anaesthesia

ANSWERS

Q1 — Pre-eclampsia

A 25-year-old woman who is 37 weeks pregnant and known to have pre-eclampsia is admitted to the labour ward with a blood pressure of 160/110mmHg on several readings.

a) What is the definition of pre-eclampsia? 1 mark

Pre-eclampsia is a multisystem disorder with:

- Hypertension (BP >140/90mmHg) presenting after 20 weeks' gestation.
- Significant proteinuria, i.e, spot urinary protein: creatinine ratio >30mg/mmol or a 24-hour urine collection with >300mg protein.

b) Define gestational hypertension. 1 mark

Hypertension presenting after 20 weeks' gestation without significant proteinuria.

c) How can you define severe pre-eclampsia? 2 marks

Proteinuria with severe hypertension (BP >160/110mmHg).
OR
Mild to moderate hypertension (140/90 to 159/109mmHg) with any of the following features:

- Severe headache.
- Visual disturbance such as flashing lights or blurring.
- Vomiting.
- Subcostal pain.
- Papilloedema.
- Clonus (≥3 beats).
- Liver tenderness.
- Thrombocytopenia (<100 × 10^9/L).
- Abnormal liver enzymes.
- HELLP syndrome.

d) Explain the pathogenesis of pre-eclampsia. 2 marks

- Impaired trophoblastic cell invasion.
- Failure of spiral artery dilatation.
- Placental hypoperfusion and hypoxia.
- Releases cytokines and inflammatory factors into the maternal circulation triggering endothelial dysfunction.
- Increase in vascular reactivity, permeability, and coagulation cascade activation.
- Organ damage.

e) Which related symptoms should pregnant women be told to report immediately? 2 marks

- Severe headache.
- Problems with vision, such as blurring or flashing before the eyes.

- Severe pain just below the ribs or abdominal pain.
- Vomiting.
- Sudden swelling of the face, hands or feet.
- Reduced foetal movement.

f) How should this patient be monitored following admission to the labour ward? 2 marks

- Obstetric consultant-led care with input from anaesthetic and neonatology teams.
- Monitor for signs and symptoms of severe pre-eclampsia.
- Monitor with the following — ECG, NIBP/IABP, pulse oximetry, RR, fluid input/output, hourly reflexes.
- Six-hourly blood tests to monitor the platelet count, renal function and liver enzymes.
- Foetal monitoring — US scan and CTG.

g) How would you control BP in this patient? 2 marks

- Maintain systolic pressure <150mmHg and diastolic pressure 80-100mmHg.
- Reduce BP at the rate of 1-2mmHg per minute.
- First-line — oral labetalol.
- Oral methyldopa and nifedipine if labetalol is contraindicated (bronchial asthma).
- Refractory hypertension — administer IV labetalol or IV hydralazine.
- Intra-arterial BP monitoring and HDU care may be considered.

h) What changes would you make to your airway management for a pregnant woman, if this woman needed a general anaesthetic for a caesarean section? 3 marks

- Anticipate a difficult airway.
- Manage the hypertensive response to laryngoscopy with alfentanil, remifentanil, esmolol, atenolol.

- Manage hypertension at emergence with the same drugs.
- Smaller size ETT due to upper airway oedema.
- Gentle airway instrumentation to avoid trauma.

i) What are the other considerations for GA? 3 mark

- Non-depolarising muscle relaxants are potentiated by magnesium sulphate; hence, smaller doses should be used with neuromuscular monitoring.
- Appropriate neonatal resuscitation facilities.
- A higher risk of PPH but avoid ergometrine.
- Good postoperative analgesia/regional techniques like TAP blocks.
- Avoid NSAIDs.
- The likelihood of postoperative airway oedema and pulmonary oedema.
- Postoperative HDU/ITU care.

j) What are the complications of pre-eclampsia? 2 mark

Maternal complications:

- Eclampsia.
- Intracerebral haemorrhage.
- Pulmonary oedema.
- Acute renal failure.
- Liver dysfunction.
- Coagulation abnormalities.

Foetal complications:

- Abruptio placentae.
- Intrauterine growth restriction.
- Premature delivery.
- Intrauterine foetal death.

References

1. Leslie D, Collis RE. Hypertension in pregnancy. *Br J Anaesth Education* 2016; 16(1): 33-72.
2. Hypertension in pregnancy: diagnosis and management. NICE clinical guideline, CG107. London: National Institute for Health and Care Excellence, 2010. https://www.nice.org.uk/guidance/cg107. Accessed on 25th June 2019.

Q2 — Postdural puncture headache

The obstetric team tell you about a patient who is 2 days postpartum with a suspicion of a postdural puncture headache (PDPH).

a) What is the differential diagnosis for this patient with a suspected postpartum headache? 3 mark

- Non-specific — dehydration, caffeine withdrawal, sleep deprivation.
- Tension headache.
- Lactation headache.
- Migraine.
- Sinusitis.
- Pre-eclampsia/eclampsia.
- Cortical vein thrombosis.
- Subarachnoid haemorrhage.
- Posterior reversible leukoencephalopathy syndrome.
- Space-occupying lesion — brain tumour, subdural haematoma.
- Cerebral infarction/ischaemia.
- Meningitis, encephalitis.

b) What features, in this patient, would lead you to consider a serious underlying cause? 3 mark

- Focal neurological deficit.
- Seizures.
- Altered conscious level.
- Absence of postural component.
- Presence of infectious markers.
- Hypertension and proteinuria — pre-eclampsia/eclampsia.

c) What is the mechanism/pathogenesis of headache in PDPH? 1 mark

CSF leakage and a decrease in intracranial pressure causes:

- Traction on unsupported intracranial pain-sensitive structures such as the tentorium and blood vessels.
- Compensatory vasodilatation of intracranial blood vessels.

d) List the clinical features of PDPH. 2 marks

- 90% of headaches develop within 3 days of the procedure.
- Headache is often frontal-occipital.
- Aggravated in the upright position, and when coughing or straining.
- Relieved on lying down.
- Associated symptoms include neck stiffness, nausea and vomiting, visual disturbance, photophobia, auditory symptoms, cranial nerve palsies.

e) List the management strategies for this patient who is suffering with a PDPH. 4 marks

- Conservative management:
  - bed rest;
  - hydration.
- Pharmacological management:
  - simple analgesia — paracetamol, NSAIDs;
  - weak opioids +/- strong opioids PRN;
  - avoid constipation — prescribe stool softeners;
  - cerebral vasoconstrictors — caffeine 800-1000mg/day = 8-10 cups of coffee.
- Epidural blood patch (EBP) — the gold standard.
- Further evidence is required before treatment with theophylline, sumatriptan, ACTH.

f) You diagnose a PDPH and arrange treatment by an epidural blood patch (EBP). How is an epidural blood patch performed? 2 marks

- Obtain consent.
- IV access.
- Complete asepsis by both anaesthetists.
- Position the patient — usually laterally for patient comfort.
- Performed at or one space below the original site of dural puncture.
- The epidural space is identified.
- The assistant should aseptically withdraw 20ml of blood from a peripheral vein.
- 10-20ml should be injected into the epidural space.
- Should radicular pain occur, slow or stop injecting.

g) What advice would you give to the patient after an EBP? 1 mark

- Post-procedure, the patient should lie flat for 1-2 hours.
- Refrain from vigorous activity or lifting for a few days.
- Consider prescribing stool softeners to avoid constipation.
- Before leaving hospital, patients should be counselled to report fever, severe back pain, or radicular pain immediately.

h) Describe the mechanism of action of an EBP. 1 mark

- Tamponade effect of blood in the epidural space.
- Increased intracranial pressure and relief from headache.
- Formation of a clot seals the puncture site preventing further CSF leak.

i) What are the described risks of an EBP? 3 marks

Risk of an epidural:

- Dural puncture.

- Permanent and temporary nerve damage.
- Meningitis.
- Risk of haematoma.

Risk of an EBP:

- Early complications:
  - backache during injection;
  - fever;
  - bradycardia;
  - seizures.
- Late complications include:
  - meningitis;
  - subdural haematoma;
  - arachnoiditis;
  - radicular pain;
  - recurrence of headache.

References

1. Sabharwal A, Stocks GM. Postpartum headache: diagnosis and management. *Br J Anaesth CEACCP* 2011; 11(5): 181-5.

Q3 — Spinal anaesthesia for a caesarean section

a) Which methods of testing may be used to confirm the adequacy of a spinal (intrathecal) block for an elective caesarean section? 6 marks

Sensory block:

- Temperature — ethyl chloride spray/cold sensation.
- Pin prick.
- Pressure.
- Touch.
- Proprioception, vibration.

A block to cold sensation at T2-4 and pin prick at T4-T5 confirms the adequacy of the block for a caesarean section.

Motor block using the Bromage scale:

- 0 = no motor block.
- 1 = inability to straight leg raise but able to move knee and feet.
- 2 = inability to straight leg raise or move knee, able to move feet.
- 3 = complete motor block.

A score of 3 indicates a higher lumbar block.

Autonomic block:

- Hypotension.
- Bradycardia.
- Temperature changes.

b) Describe the actions you could take if your spinal block proves inadequate on testing prior to starting surgery for an elective (category 4) caesarean section. 3 marks

- Tilting the patient head down.
- If there is no evidence of block after 20 minutes, repeat the same dose of spinal or do a combined spinal epidural.
- If the block is inadequate, consider an epidural catheter and gradual top-ups. Repeating the spinal in this case may lead to a high/total spinal.
- Consider GA.
- Discussion with the mother, surgeon and senior colleague, and foetal monitoring to influence decision-making.

c) What are the early symptoms and signs of a spinal block that is ascending too high? 5 marks

T1-T4 block:

- Weak cough, shortness of breath (paralysis of intercoastal muscles).
- Hypotension and bradycardia (cardiac sympathetic block).
- Nausea and vomiting.
- Foetal compromise.

C6-C8 block:

- Paraesthesia of hands and arms.

C3-C5 block:

- Desaturation and respiratory arrest (diaphragmatic paralysis).
- Brainstem involvement and intracranial spread:
  - a difficulty in phonation and swallowing;
  - loss of consciousness.

d) How should you manage a patient who complains of pain during an elective caesarean section under spinal anaesthesia? 6 marks

- Stop surgery if required.
- Reassure.
- Communication with the mother and surgeon.
- Offer analgesia.
- Entonox®.
- Intravenous opioid:
  - 25-50μg fentanyl, repeat as necessary;
  - inform the neonatologist if this is given before delivery of the baby.
- Surgical infiltration of local anaesthetic.
- Epidural opioid/LA.
- General anaesthesia.

References

1. Fettes PDW, Jansson J-R, Wildsmith JAW. Failed spinal anaesthesia: mechanisms, management, and prevention. *Br J Anaesth* 2009; 102(6): 739-48.
2. Allman K, Wilson I, O'Donnell A, Eds. *Oxford Handbook of Anaesthesia*, 4th ed. Oxford: Oxford University Press, 2016.

Q4 — Intrauterine foetal death

A woman, who has had an intrauterine foetal death (IUFD) at 36 weeks' gestation in her first pregnancy, is admitted to the delivery suite for induction of labour.

a) List the causes of IUFD. 4 marks

Antepartum:

- Congenital malformation.
- APH.
- Pre-eclampsia/eclampsia.
- Maternal diabetes mellitus.

Intrapartum:

- Abruptio placentae.
- Severe maternal or foetal infection.
- Cord prolapse.
- Uterine rupture.

b) Describe the important non-clinical aspects of her management. 3 marks

- Psychological distress needs to be addressed.
- One-to-one midwifery care.
- Care provided in a quiet room.
- Free access to family members if the mother wishes.
- Pain relief options to be discussed by an anaesthetist.
- May require HDU care.

c) What are the considerations when providing pain relief for this woman prior to delivery? 5 marks

Patient factors:

- Address psychological distress.
- Consider pre-existing comorbidities.
- Sepsis.
- Coagulopathy.

Obstetric factors:

- Cause of IUFD.
- Mode of delivery:
  - early induction of labour;
  - may require a caesarean section.

Others:

- One-to-one midwifery care.
- MEOWS charting.
- May require HDU care.
- Consider sedation.

d) What are the options for pain relief? 4 marks

- Entonox®.
- Parenteral opioids — diamorphine/pethidine IM, morphine/fentanyl/remifentanil PCA.
- Supplementary regular IV/oral paracetamol.
- Regional anaesthesia with epidural PCEA — if not contraindicated.

e) If this patient requires a caesarean section what are the advantages of using regional anaesthesia, other than the avoidance of the effects of general anaesthesia? 4 marks

- Good postoperative analgesia.
- Early mobilisation.
- Decreased risk of PPH.
- Decreased risk of DVT.
- Fewer drugs — less chance of anaphylaxis and drowsiness.

References

1. Late intrauterine fetal death and stillbirth. Green-top guideline, no. 55. London: Royal College of Obstetrics and Gynaecology. https://www.rcog.org.uk/en/guidelines-research-services/guidelines /gtg55/. Accessed on 25th June 2019.
2. Allman K, Wilson I, O'Donnell A, Eds. *Oxford Handbook of Anaesthesia*, 4th ed. Oxford: Oxford University Press, 2016.

Q5 — Obesity and pregnancy

A primiparous patient with a BMI of 55kg/m^2 presents in the high-risk anaesthetic antenatal assessment clinic at 34 weeks' gestation. She is hoping to have a normal delivery.

a) What are the specific cardiorespiratory effects of obesity in the pregnant patient? 4 marks

Cardiovascular system:

- Increase in stroke volume, heart rate, and increased pulse pressure associated with pregnancy may be poorly tolerated.
- Hypertension, ischaemic heart disease and congestive heart failure.
- Exaggerated response to aortocaval compression due to increased intra-abdominal fat.
- Peripartum cardiomyopathy.

Respiratory system:

- Decrease in FRC associated with normal pregnancy is aggravated.
- Postoperative hypoxia and atelectasis.
- Obstructive sleep apnoea.
- Pulmonary hypertension and cor pulmonale.
- Restrictive respiratory pattern.

b) What are the specific obstetric concerns associated with a raised BMI in pregnancy? 3 marks

Increased risks of:

- Gestational DM, PIH, pre-eclampsia.
- Thromboembolic disorders.
- Instrumental and caesarean delivery.

- Postpartum haemorrhage.
- Postoperative infections (surgical wound and chest infections).
- Peripartum cardiomyopathy.

c) What are the foetal risks associated with a high BMI? 3 marks

Increased risks of:

- Miscarriage, preterm birth, still birth.
- Meconium aspiration.
- Foetal distress.
- Shoulder dystocia.
- Neural tube defects, macrosomia.
- Low Apgar score.
- A higher incidence of neonatal intensive care admissions.

d) What are your anaesthetic concerns in this obstetric patient with a high BMI? 6 marks

- Difficult intravenous access.
- Difficulty performing neuraxial techniques and a high risk of dural puncture.
- A higher incidence of failed blocks due to altered spread of LA secondary to fat deposition in the epidural space.
- Risks with GA:
  - difficult airway;
  - risk of aspiration;
  - short apnoea time due to decreased FRC and increased oxygen consumption;
  - increased oxygen requirements postoperatively.
- Equipment issues and staff:
  - maximum weight supported by operating table;
  - risk to staff involved in manual handling;
  - longer spinal and epidural needles;

- larger BP cuffs, TEDs, Flowtron®;
- US for venous access, arterial and central venous cannulation.

e) What are your considerations when you provide labour analgesia? 4 marks

- Review of antenatal consultation notes with obstetric anaesthetist.
- Difficult IV access.
- Early epidural to allow time for a difficult procedure.
- US scan of the back to facilitate epidural insertion.
- Supplemental analgesia with Entonox® and oral/IV paracetamol.
- Analgesic options in the case of a failed epidural — remifentanil/fentanyl PCA.
- If opioids are used, supplemental oxygen, pulse oximetry and one-to-one midwifery care is needed.

References

1. Gupta A, Faber P. Obesity in pregnancy. *Br J Anaesth CEACCP* 2011; 11(4): 143-6.

Q6 — Surgery in pregnancy

A 28-year-old woman presents for an acute appendicectomy under general anaesthesia; she is 22 weeks pregnant.

a) List the risks to the foetus during anaesthesia in this situation. 4 marks

- Spontaneous abortion.
- Preterm labour.
- IUGR.
- Foetal death.
- Placental ischaemia and foetal hypoxia.
- Foetal acidosis/ion trapping and myocardial depression.
- Teratogenicity in the first trimester.

b) How can the risks to the foetus be minimised? 2 marks

- Timing of surgery.
- Avoid foetal hypoxia.
- Prevention of preterm labour.
- Consider the effects of anaesthetic drugs on the foetus.

c) How does timing the surgery reduce the foetal risk? 1 mark

- Elective surgeries to be postponed at least 6 weeks postpartum, if possible.
- Alternatively, delay surgeries into the second trimester to avoid the teratogenic effects of drugs.

d) What steps would you take to avoid foetal hypoxia? 5 marks

- Avoid maternal hypoxia:
  - adequate pre-oxygenation;

- anti-aspiration prophylaxis;
- RSI.

- Maintain maternal haemodynamic stability.
- Avoid maternal hypocapnia and hypercapnia (maintain $PaCO_2$ around 4kPa):
  - hypocapnia causes placental vasoconstriction;
  - hypercapnia decreases the transfer of CO_2 from the foetus to the mother across the placental barrier, causing foetal acidosis.
- Avoid hypovolaemia and anaemia.
- Light planes of anaesthesia increase catecholamine secretion — placental vasoconstriction and hypoperfusion.
- Effective postoperative analgesia — pain causes placental vasoconstriction and foetal hypoxia.
- Detection and suppression of premature labour with tocolytics.

e) List any four drugs used in anaesthetic practice and their adverse effects on the foetus. 4 marks

- Ketamine increases uterine tone and vasoconstriction in the first two trimesters.
- NSAIDs in the third trimester cause closure of the ductus arteriosus.
- Nitrous oxide interferes with DNA synthesis.
- Single-dose opioids and benzodiazepines are safe. Long-term use causes withdrawal when the foetus is delivered.

f) What additional preoperative and intraoperative steps would you take to ensure foetal safety if she is 27 weeks pregnant instead? 4 marks

The foetus is viable as it is at 27 weeks' gestation.

Preoperatively:

- Discussion with the obstetric team to plan for preterm labour and delivery.

- Discussion with paediatricians/PICU.
- Consider steroids for lung maturation.
- FHR and FHR variability monitoring. FHR variability is observed from 25 weeks onwards.
- CTG monitoring preoperatively and postoperatively.

Intraoperatively:

- The physiological effects of pregnancy may be more pronounced.
- The presence of obstetricians/midwife on site.

References

1. Nejdlova M, Johnson T. Anaesthesia for non-obstetric procedures during pregnancy. *Br J Anaesth CEACCP* 2012; 12(4): 203-6.

Q7 — Airway problems in pregnancy

a) What factors may contribute to difficulties encountered when securing the airway under general anaesthesia in the pregnant patient? 9 marks

Obstetric factors:

- Decreased FRC and increased oxygen consumption — decreases the safe apnoea time.
- Increased weight gain, large breasts — difficult laryngoscopy.
- Airway oedema — a smaller-sized ETT may be required.
- Increased vascularity of the mucosa — bleeding on airway instrumentation.
- High risk of aspiration.

Human factors:

- Cognitive load — concerns for mother and baby.
- Time restrictions — often an emergency situation.
- Declining frequency of obstetric GA.

Technical factors:

- Remote location of obstetric units.
- Poor access to the airway under the drapes.
- Misplaced cricoid pressure.

b) What measures can be taken to reduce airway-related morbidity and mortality associated with general anaesthesia in a pregnant woman? 8 marks

- Assessment of the airway.
- Identify senior help and call for help early.

- Mark the cricothyroid membrane and call for surgical help if a difficulty is anticipated.
- Adequate pre-oxygenation — 3-4 minutes of tidal breathing or 4-5 vital capacity breaths.
- Ramped up position — tragus in line with or above the sternal notch.
- Apnoeic oxygenation.
- Anti-aspiration prophylaxis.
- Training staff to be familiar with the Difficult Airway Society (DAS) guidelines.
- Multidisciplinary team briefing with regard to waking up the patient or not after a failed intubation is declared.

c) What are the recommendations in the 4th National Audit Project (Major Complications of Airway Management in the UK, NAP4) regarding airway management in the pregnant woman? 3 marks

- Obstetric anaesthetists to maintain airway skills including a difficult/failed intubation and CICV.
- Anaesthetists to be familiar and skilled with rescue second-generation supraglottic airway devices (SADs).
- Department to provide skills and equipment to deliver AFOI whenever it is needed.
- All staff in the recovery area of a delivery suite must be competency trained; skills to be regularly updated.

References

1. Major complications of airway management in the United Kingdom NAP4. National Audit Project, 2011. https://www.rcoa.ac.uk/system/files/CSQ-NAP4-Full.pdf. Accessed on 25th June 2019.
2. DAS guidelines. Guidelines for the management of difficult and failed tracheal intubation in obstetrics. Difficult Airway Society, 2015. https://das.uk.com/guidelines/obstetric_airway_guidelines_2015. Accessed on 25th June 2019.
3. Mushambi MC, Kinsella SM, Popat M, *et al*. Obstetric Anaesthetist's Association and Difficult Airway Society guidelines for the management of difficult and failed tracheal intubation in obstetrics. *Anaesthesia* 2015; 70(11): 1286-306

Q8 — Mitral stenosis in pregnancy

A 27-year-old woman is 13 weeks pregnant. In the antenatal clinic she is found to have an asymptomatic heart murmur. A subsequent echocardiogram shows moderate to severe mitral stenosis.

a) List the causes of mitral stenosis (MS). 2 mar

- Rheumatic heart disease.
- Congenital.
- Diseases affecting multiple systems, e.g. sarcoidosis.
- Infiltrating diseases.

b) What are the echocardiographic criteria for the diagnosis of severity of MS? 2 mar

Mitral stenosis is classified as per:

- Valve area:
  - mild MS — 1.6-2cm^2;
  - moderate MS — 1.5-1cm^2;
  - severe MS — <1cm^2.
- Pressure gradients across the valve:
  - mild MS — <5mmHg;
  - moderate MS — 6-10mmHg;
  - severe MS — >10mmHg.

c) What is the normal mitral valve area and at what point does the patient become symptomatic with MS? 2 mar

- Normal area = 4-6cm^2.
- The patient becomes symptomatic at a valve area <2cm^2.

d) What are the cardiovascular changes in pregnancy that could exacerbate the pathophysiology of MS? 3 marks

- Increase in heart rate.
- Increased cardiac output.
- Blood volume increases.
- Decreased systemic vascular resistance.
- Pain and anxiety in labour further increase cardiac output.
- Autotransfusion during the second stage.

e) How do the cardiovascular changes in pregnancy exacerbate the pathophysiology of MS? 3 marks

- Mitral stenosis underfills the left ventricle causing pressure and volume overload in the pulmonary circulation. Tachycardia of pregnancy decreases diastolic filling time, further decreasing left ventricular filling, increases pulmonary pressures causing pulmonary congestion. Pulmonary oedema can develop with AF.
- The fixed cardiac output state of MS results in a worsening of pressure through the pulmonary circulation and into the right heart.
- Increased blood volume of pregnancy increases preload and exacerbates pulmonary oedema.
- Because the cardiac output is fixed, any decrease in systemic vascular resistance decreases the coronary perfusion pressures.
- The risk of decompensation depends on severity. Anything worse than moderate disease (valve area $<1.5cm^2$) frequently results in heart failure, which usually develops in the second or third trimester and is progressive.

f) What are your cardiovascular goals when she presents in labour? 2 marks

- Control of rate and rhythm:
  - avoid tachycardia;
  - avoid a rapid ventricular response in AF.

- Maintain afterload.
- Avoid an increase in preload.
- Avoid hypoxia, hypercarbia and acidosis as they exacerbate pulmonary hypertension.

g) Outline your management of this patient in labour. 5 mar

- Early epidural to avoid sympathetic stimulation.
- Establishment of a block gradually to avoid precipitous hypotension.
- Use of alpha-agonists to treat hypotension.
- Nitrous oxide increases pulmonary vascular resistance.
- Assist the second stage to cut short labour and limit the Valsalva manoeuvre.
- Caution with oxytocin as it decreases SVR and increases PVR.
- Ergometrine is contraindicated as it is a pulmonary vasoconstrictor.

h) Explain the mechanism of pulmonary oedema post-delivery. 1 mar

A sudden increase in preload due to:

- Autotransfusion due to uterine contraction.
- Decompression of the IVC.

References

1. Holmes K, Gibbison B, Vohra HA. Mitral valve and mitral valve disease. *Br J Anaesth Education* 2017; 17(1): 1-9.

Q9 — Amniotic fluid embolism

A 39-year-old multiparous woman is admitted post-term with spontaneous rupture of membranes and meconium-stained liquor. After an epidural catheter is inserted, a syntocinon infusion is started as she is in early labour. She started contracting shortly and the foetal heart rate drops. She becomes breathless and cyanosed; her blood pressure has dropped.

a) What are the differential diagnoses for this presentation? 6 marks

Obstetric causes:

- Amniotic fluid embolism.
- Uterine rupture.
- Eclampsia.
- Placental abruption.
- Acute haemorrhage.
- Cardiomyopathy.
- Uterine inversion.

Non-obstetric causes:

- Pulmonary embolism.
- Air or fat embolism.
- Tension pneumothorax.
- Anaphylaxis.
- High spinal/epidural, local anaesthetic toxicity.
- Pulmonary oedema, heart failure, myocardial infarction.
- Sepsis.
- Transfusion reaction.
- Aspiration.

- Respiratory condition exacerbation.
- Intracranial bleed.

b) What are the risk factors for an amniotic fluid embolism (AFE)? 2 mar

- Induction of labour by any method.
- Use of oxytocin.
- Assisted delivery (forceps/ventouse) or caesarean section.
- Maternal age >35 years.
- Multiple pregnancy.
- Polyhydramnios.
- Eclampsia.
- Uterine rupture.
- Cervical trauma.
- Placenta praevia.
- Placental abruption.
- Ethnic minority.

c) Describe the pathogenesis of AFE. 2 mar

- Exposure of maternal circulation to amniotic fluid or foetal antigens is a prerequisite.
- There are two main theories — mechanical and immune-mediated.
- Anaphylactoid syndrome.
- Phase 1 — lasts 30 minutes, entry of amniotic fluid into the circulation, the pulmonary artery pressure rises, right ventricular failure, microvascular damage, hypotension. Microthrombi are formed once DIC develops.
- Phase 2 — left ventricular failure, endothelial activation and leakage, leading to DIC.

d) What are the clinical features of AFE? 4 mar

- Hypotension and foetal distress are identified in all cases of AFE.
- Sudden cardiovascular collapse or cardiac arrest.

- Cyanosis, dyspnoea, seizures, coagulopathy, pulmonary oedema, ARDS.
- Uterine atony, bronchospasm, cough, headache, chest pain.

e) How would you diagnose AFE? 2 marks

- Clinical symptoms once other causes are ruled out.
- Postmortem — foetal squames or hair in lungs.

f) What is the incidence of AFE? 1 mark

- 1.7 per 100,000 pregnancies.
- The case fatality is 19%.
- 120 cases between 2005 and 2014; UKOSS register.
- Fifth direct cause of maternal mortality (MBRRACE-UK report).

g) List the management strategies for AFE. 3 marks

Supportive management depending on the clinical presentation:

- Senior clinicians should be involved, teamwork, urgent decision to deliver, need for critical care support.
- Advanced Life Support® guidelines — ABC.
- Haemorrhage control.
- Coagulation abnormalities to be corrected; involve the senior haematology consultant.

References

1. Metodiev Y, Ramasamy P, Tuffnell D. Amniotic fluid embolism. *Br J Anaesth Education* 2018; 18(8): 234-8.

Q10 — Labour analgesia and puerperal sepsis

a) Describe the pain pathways associated with the first and second stages of labour. 2 marks

- The first stage of labour: pain from the uterus, lower uterine segment and vagina is transmitted via sensory fibres which accompany sympathetic nerves and ends in the dorsal horns of T10-L1.
- The second stage of labour: afferent nerves innervating the vagina and perineum travel via the pudendal nerve to dorsal root ganglia of S2-S4.

b) Explain how and why the nature of the pain experienced changes as labour progresses. 2 marks

- The first stage of labour: visceral pain, which is poorly localised and diffuse in nature.
- Pain is felt in the lower abdomen and lumbosacral area.
- The second stage of labour: somatic pain, which is better localised.

c) What dermatomes should be blocked for labour analgesia and a lower segment caesarean section (LSCS)? 2 marks

- Labour analgesia — T10-S5.
- LSCS — T4-S5.

d) Why is it essential to achieve a higher dermatomal level of regional block for a caesarean section than for analgesia in labour? 1 mark

A higher level of block is required for LSCSs — due to peritoneal traction.

e) Why do you sometimes observe bradycardia during regional anaesthesia for a caesarean section? 2 marks

- Parasympathetic over-activity due to spinal sympathetic block.
- Decreased venous return triggers the Bainbridge reflex and Bezold-Jarisch reflex.
- Blockade of cardio-accelerator fibres from T1-T4.
- Surgical manoeuvres, e.g. exteriorising the uterus.

f) List any five specific situations in which labour epidurals may be beneficial. 4 marks

- Pre-eclampsia (without severe thrombocytopenia or coagulopathy).
- High Body Mass Index (BMI).
- Anticipated difficult airway or other risk factors for a general anaesthetic.
- High risk for assisted vaginal delivery, e.g. breech or multiple gestation.
- Trial of labour after a previous caesarean section.
- Maternal cardiovascular, cerebrovascular or respiratory disease.

g) What is puerperal sepsis? 2 marks

Puerperal sepsis is infection of the genital tract occurring at any time between rupture of membranes or labour and the 42nd day postpartum associated with two or more of the following:

- Pelvic pain.
- Fever, abnormal vaginal discharge.
- Abnormal smell of discharge.
- Delay in reduction in the size of the uterus.

h) Name the organisms implicated in sepsis in the UK. 2 marks

- Group A *Streptococcus*.
- *Streptococcus pneumoniae*.
- *Escherichia coli*.
- H1N1 influenza virus.

i) List the risk factors for sepsis. 3 marks

Obstetric factors:

- During pregnancy:
  - amniocentesis;
  - cervical suture.
- During vaginal delivery:
  - prolonged rupture of membranes;
  - prolonged labour;
  - vaginal trauma;
  - surgical procedures — episiotomy, caesarean section;
  - retained products.

Non-obstetric factors:

- Obesity.
- Diabetes.
- Immunosuppression.
- Anaemia.
- Socioeconomic deprivation.
- History of pelvic inflammatory disease.

References

1. Elton RJ, Chaudhari S. Sepsis in obstetrics. *Br J Anaesth CEACCP* 2015; 15(5): 259-64.
2. Allman K, Wilson I, O'Donnell A, Eds. *Oxford Handbook of Anaesthesia*, 4th ed. Oxford: Oxford University Press, 2016.

Chapter 13

Paediatric anaesthesia

ANSWERS

Q1 — Down's syndrome

A 9-year-old child is listed for a dental extraction in a day-case list.

a) List the cardiovascular problems in Down's syndrome relevant to an anaesthetist. 2 marks

- Congenital heart diseases — atrioventricular canal defects, ASD, VSD, TOF.
- Pulmonary hypertension secondary to a left to right shunt.
- Cardiac conduction defects are likely following repairs if there is congenital heart disease.

b) List the airway/respiratory problems in Down's syndrome of relevance to the anaesthetist. 5 marks

- Obstructive sleep apnoea — secondary to craniofacial abnormalities.
- Likely difficult airway — secondary to macroglossia, narrow midface, oropharyngeal hypotonia, micrognathia, small mouth, short neck, adenotonsillar hypertrophy.
- Tracheal and subglottic stenosis — 2-6% cases.
- Prone to recurrent lower respiratory tract infection.
- Gastro-oesophageal reflux — aspiration risk.

c) List the neurological problems that are associated with this syndrome in children and its relevance to the anaesthetist. 3 mark

- Developmental delay — communication issues with ocular and acoustic impairments.
- Intellectual impairment — agitation in the postoperative period.
- Generalised hypotonia and joint laxity — positioning-related nerve damage.
- Epilepsy and antiepileptic medication implications.
- A higher risk of sedation and respiratory depression with opiates.

d) What are the potential problems during induction of anaesthesia and the initial airway management in this patient? 6 marks

- Cannulation may be difficult.
- Communication difficulties can lead to an anxious and uncooperative child.
- Anxious parents.
- The possibility of a difficult airway due to craniofacial abnormalities.
- Aspiration risk due to gastro-oesophageal reflux.
- Atlanto-axial instability — chances of spinal cord compression with neck movements.
- A smaller sized ETT may be needed due to subglottic stenosis and tracheal stenosis.

e) What are the possible specific difficulties in the postoperative management of this child? 4 mark

- Communication issues.
- A higher likelihood for agitation.
- Pain assessment and management are difficult.
- Prone to side effects such as sedation, airway obstruction and respiratory depression from anaesthetic drugs including opioids.

References

1. Short JA, Calder A. Anaesthesia for children with special needs, including autistic spectrum disorder. *Br J Anaesth CEACCP* 2013; 13(4): 107-12.
2. Allt JE, Howell CJ. Down's syndrome. *Br J Anaesth CEPD Reviews* 2003; 3(3): 83-6.

Q2 — Day-case eye surgery

A 4-year-old boy is listed for elective strabismus surgery in a day-case ophthalmology theatre list.

a) List the anaesthetic considerations for this patient with regards to his age. 4 marks

- Establish communication with parents and child.
- He may need topical analgesia (e.g. Ametop® cream, EMLA cream) for IV access.
- Associated chromosomal and metabolic conditions need to be ruled out in this child.
- Associated anomalies, if present, need addressing — mental retardation, behavioural problems and delayed development.
- Associated syndromes with craniofacial involvement, e.g. Goldenhar syndrome, Treacher Collins, etc., can pose airway difficulties.
- Associated conditions such as seizures and congenital cardiac abnormalities need managing appropriately.

b) List the anaesthetic considerations of this case with regards to day-case surgery. 3 marks

- A high incidence of postoperative nausea and vomiting — unplanned overnight admission.
- Pain management challenges in children with communication difficulties.
- The child may need observation overnight if he is associated with developmental delay and mental retardation in view of the likelihood of respiratory depression and airway obstruction postoperatively.

c) List the anaesthetic considerations with regards to strabismus surgery. **4 marks**

- Limited access to the airway which needs to be secured well, e.g. a reinforced endotracheal tube can be taped well and all the connections in the anaesthetic circuit need to be well secured.
- Associated with an oculocardiac reflex secondary to extraocular muscle traction.
- A higher incidence of malignant hyperthermia (MH) in squint surgeries.
- May need to avoid suxamethonium — to minimise the risk of increased (extraocular) muscle tone and MH.
- Avoid muscle relaxants if botulinum toxin is planned to be injected into the extraocular muscles by the surgeon.
- Anti-sickness prophylaxis intraoperatively — the use of 5-HT3 antagonists, e.g. ondansetron, are effective.

d) During the operation, the patient suddenly develops a profound bradycardia. What is your immediate management of this situation? **2 marks**

- This is likely due to an oculocardiac reflex.
- IV atropine 20μg/kg followed by IV normal saline as a flush.
- Inform the surgeon about bradycardia and to stop the surgical stimulation of extraocular muscles.

e) What strategies would you employ to reduce postoperative nausea and vomiting (PONV) in this patient? **4 marks**

- 5-HT3 antagonist, e.g. IV ondansetron 0.1mg/kg.
- Combination therapy of ondansetron with IV dexamethasone 0.15mg/kg.
- Total intravenous anaesthesia can be used to reduce PONV.

- Other drugs such as IV droperidol 0.025mg/kg may be given in established nausea and vomiting.
- Avoid dehydration.
- Avoid nitrous oxide.
- Minimise the use of opiods in the postoperative period by opioid-sparing analgesics.
- Minimise the use of anticholinesterase drugs for the reversal of non-depolarising muscle relaxants (NDMRs) by avoiding the use of NDMRs.

f) What strategies would you employ to reduce postoperative pain in this child? 3 marks

- Multimodal analgesia.
- Local anaesthetic infiltration intraoperatively, e.g. subtenon's block.
- Paracetamol 15mg/kg QDS.
- NSAID, e.g. rectal suppository of diclofenac 12.5mg BD to TDS.
- Minimise/avoid the use of intraoperative opioids.

References

1. James I. Anaesthesia for paediatric eye surgery. *Br J Anaesth CEACCP* 2008; 8(1): 5-10.

Q3 — Meningococcal sepsis

You are called to the emergency department to see a 2-year-old child who presents with a 4-hour history of high temperature and drowsiness. On examination, there is a prolonged capillary refill time and a non-blanching rash. A presumptive diagnosis of meningococcal septicaemia is made.

a) What is the normal weight, pulse rate, systolic arterial blood pressure and capillary refill time for a child of this age? 4 marks

For a 2-year-old child:

- Normal weight = 2 x Age +8 = 2 x 2 + 8 = 12kg.
- Pulse rate = around 95 to 140/minute.
- Systolic arterial blood pressure = 85 to 100mmHg.
- Capillary refill time <2 seconds.

b) Define appropriate resuscitation goals for this child. 2 marks

Goals:

- Early treatment of septicaemia.
- Haemodynamic resuscitation.
- Correct metabolic disturbances, e.g. hypokalaemia, hypoglycaemia, acidosis.
- Correct coagulopathy.

c) Outline the management in the first 15 minutes after presentation. 6 marks

- Call for help.
- ABCD approach and stabilisation.
- Blood gas.

- Oxygen supplementation — using a reservoir rebreathing mask at 15L/min O_2.
- Early IV antibiotics according to local policy — first choice: IV ceftriaxone.
- Fluid resuscitation with crystalloids — 20ml/kg of 0.9% normal saline IV fluid bolus over 5-10 minutes — to be repeated if needed.
- If signs of shock persist after 40ml/kg of normal saline — inform the paediatric intensivist.
- IV human albumin 4.5% can also be administered instead of a second bolus of normal saline.
- Vasopressors if shock persists after fluid boluses — IV infusion of noradrenaline or adrenaline.
- If there is respiratory failure or decreasing consciousness — airway support with tracheal intubation (ideally by a paediatric anaesthetist) and mechanical ventilation, with transfer to the paediatric intensive care if there is airway compromise.
- Control of seizures if needed.

d) After 15 minutes, the child remains shocked and is unresponsive to fluid. What is the most likely pathophysiological derangement in this child's circulation? 2 marks

Severe metabolic acidosis likely due to intravascular fluid depletion.

e) What are the important further treatment options in this case after the first 15 to 20 minutes? 6 marks

- Further investigations — blood culture, full blood count, CRP, blood gas, clotting screen, blood glucose, blood PCR for *Neisseria meningitidis*.
- Lumbar puncture for CSF analysis — correct coagulation if needed first.
- Liaise with the paediatric intensive care unit (PICU) team for brain imaging and transfer.

- Maintenance IV fluids along with urine output monitoring.
- Continue vasopressor infusions as needed, e.g. adrenaline or noradrenaline infusion.
- Steroid supplementation (low dose) if shock is resistant to vasopressors — hydrocortisone 25mg/m^2 body surface area QDS as directed by the PICU team.
- Correct metabolic disturbances as indicated — hypokalaemia, hypoglycaemia, acidosis, hypocalcaemia.
- Plan to correct coagulopathy and anaemia with blood and blood products as needed.
- Notify the local authorities as appropriate.

References

1. Bacterial meningitis and meningococcal septicaemia in under 16s overview. NICE clinical guideline, CG102. London: National Institute for Health and Care Excellence, 2015. https://pathways.nice.org.uk/pathways/bacterial-meningitis-and-meningococcal-septicaemia-in-under-16s. Accessed on 25th June 2019.

Q4 — Hernia repair in preterm babies

A 12-week-old male baby presents for a unilateral inguinal hernia repair. He was born at 30 weeks' gestation (30/40).

a) What are the airway and respiratory concerns in this baby? 5 mark

Airway:

- Narrow subglottis.
- Compliant trachea — more prone to malacia.
- Short trachea — prone to endobronchial intubation.

Respiratory system:

- May have bronchopulmonary dysplasia (may need a longer expiratory time on the ventilator settings, to avoid trauma).
- A higher risk of postoperative apnoea (needs postoperative apnoea monitoring).
- Possible inaccuracies in the gas volumes delivered and measured can cause trauma to the incompletely formed lungs.
- Inadequate ventilation owing to breathing circuit dead space and compliance.

b) What are the circulatory and metabolic concerns in this patient? 5 marks

Cardiovascular system:

- Persistent foetal circulation leads to shunting of blood:
  - patent intracardiac communications (foramen ovale);
  - patent extracardiac communications (ductus arteriosus).

- Stiff non-compliant ventricles with rate-dependent cardiac output:
  - heart rate fluctuations — poorly tolerated.
- Low pulmonary vascular resistance:
  - any rise in pulmonary vascular resistance will lead to worsening of right to left shunting with resultant hypoxia.

Fluids and electrolytes issues:

- Increased transepidermal fluid loss and insensible fluid loss:
  - reduce the preoperative fasting duration to 2 hours for clear fluids.
- Immature renal tubular function:
  - risk of hyponatraemia.

c) What oxygen saturation range would you aim to achieve in this patient and why? 2 marks

- Use preductal oxygen saturations with a target of 91-95%.
- Oxygen toxicity risk due to immature oxidative systems.

d) List four other possible major morbidities that could be associated in this child. 2 marks

- Respiratory distress syndrome.
- Retinopathy of prematurity — may be worsened by oxygen toxicity.
- Necrotising enterocolitis.
- Intraventricular haemorrhage.
- Sepsis.

e) What are the advantages of general anaesthesia for this baby? 3 marks

- Widely accepted technique.
- Can be supplemented with a regional analgesia technique such as a caudal epidural technique for better postoperative analgesia.

- There is no time restriction unlike central neuraxial blockade with an awake spinal for surgical time.

f) What are the disadvantages of general anaesthesia for this baby? 3 mark

- Increased intra-abdominal pressure during laproscopic surgery can limit diaphragmatic excursions; ventilation could be compromised if this is combined with CO_2 insufflation.
- A risk of respiratory complications, e.g. tracheal tube dislodgement.
- Reduced venous return causing reflex tachycardia — poorly tolerated in the presence of intravascular fluid depletion.
- A pulmonary hypertensive crisis precipitated by hypoxia/hypercarbia/acidosis can cause a right to left shunt.
- A gas embolism risk in CO_2 insufflation causing paradoxical embolus.
- The potential for neurotoxicity with exposure to general anaesthetics — neuronal apoptosis.
- A high risk of postoperative apnoea.

References

1. Ahmad N, Greenaway S. Anaesthesia for inguinal hernia repair in the newborn or ex-premature infant. *Br J Anaesth Education* 2018; 18(7): 211-7.

Q5 — Upper respiratory infection and anaesthesia

A 5-year-old boy presents for a myringotomy and grommet insertion as a day case. During your preoperative assessment you notice that he has nasal discharge.

a) Why would it be inappropriate to cancel the operation with this information? 1 mark

- The runny nose could be benign and non-infectious.
- A thorough history, examination and evaluation of other factors are needed.

b) What are the potential anaesthetic problems in a child with upper respiratory tract infection? 4 marks

- Breath-holding.
- Laryngospasm.
- Bronchospasm.
- Desaturation in the perioperative period.

c) List five features in the history that would potentially cause an increased risk of airway complications. 5 marks

- Productive cough.
- Pyrexia.
- Dyspnoea.
- Malaise.
- Irritability.
- History of asthma.
- Current or recent antibiotic therapy.
- Parental smoking.

d) List five features in the examination that would potentially cause an increased risk of airway complications. 5 marks

- Flaring of nostrils.
- Purulent nasal discharge.
- Temperature >38°C.
- Bronchial breathing.
- Wheeze.
- Crackles.
- Enlarged tonsils.

e) What perioperative airway factors would you consider in decision-making? 2 marks

- Avoid airway irritation.
- A tracheal tube is required.

f) What social factors would prevent this child being treated as a day case? 3 marks

- The lack of a responsible adult to stay and care for the child.
- The lack of access to a telephone and transport.
- Living too far away.

References

1. Bhatia N, Barber N. Dilemmas in the preoperative assessment of children. *Br J Anaesth CEACCP* 2011; 11(6): 214-8.
2. Miller RD, Ed. *Anesthesia*, 8th ed. Philadelphia: Churchill Livingstone Elsevier, 2014.
3. Butterworth JF IV, Mackey DC, Wasnick JD. *Morgan and Mikhail's Clinical Anesthesiology*, 6th ed. New York: McGraw Hill, 2018.

Q6 — Foreign body inhalation in a child

An 8-year-old girl is suspected to have inhaled a plastic bead while playing. She looks frightened, is coughing, has an audible stridor and is saturating 96% on room air.

a) List any three possible complications from foreign body inhalation. 3 marks

- Direct trauma from the foreign body.
- Airway irritation.
- Partial or complete obstruction.
- Hypoxia.
- Undetected foreign body leading to lung collapse.
- Undetected foreign body leading to recurrent chest infections.

b) What are the main features in the preoperative assessment of a child who has an inhaled foreign body? 5 marks

- Develop rapport with the child.
- Thorough assessment of the child:
  - last meal;
  - past medical history;
  - history of medications;
  - allergies;
  - previous anaesthetic history;
  - family history of any anaesthetic problems.
- Assess airway.
- Investigations and imaging as needed (CXR may not show the foreign body).
- Assess the need for sedation.
- Consider anticholinergic premedication.
- Discuss parental presence during the induction.

c) What are the main challenges during surgery for foreign body retrieval from the airway? 4 mar

- Shared airway.
- Possibility of complete airway obstruction.
- Airway trauma.
- Fragmentation of the foreign body.
- Laryngospasm and bronchospasm.
- Risk of barotrauma with positive pressure ventilation (ball valve obstruction).

d) What are the key goals of intraoperative anaesthetic conduct? 6 mar

- Ensure a patent airway.
- Good rapport with the surgeon.
- Adequate depth of anaesthesia.
- Try to preserve spontaneous ventilation.
- If positive pressure ventilation is chosen, avoid pushing the foreign body further in and causing complete airway obstruction.
- Inhalational or gaseous induction.
- Topical anaesthesia of airway.
- Maintain oxygenation.
- Insufflate or jet ventilate through a rigid bronchoscope.
- Ensure a good airway patency at emergence from anaesthesia.

e) What postoperative measures could help in a suspected traumatic bronchoscopy? 2 mark

- Steroids.
- Adrenaline nebulisation.
- Bronchodilators.
- Consider elective ventilation until the oedema subsides.

References

1. Roberts S, Thornington RE. Paediatric bronchoscopy. *Br J Anaesth CEACCP* 2005; 5(2): 41-4.
2. Bould MD. Essential notes: the anaesthetic management of an inhaled foreign body in a child. *Br J Anaesth Education* 2019; 19(3): 66-7.
3. Allman K, Wilson I, O'Donnell A, Eds. *Oxford Handbook of Anaesthesia*, 4th ed. Oxford: Oxford University Press, 2016.

Q7 — Congenital diaphragmatic hernia

A 31-year-old primiparous lady had an emergency caesarean section for foetal distress. You are the anaesthetist and deliver her by general anaesthesia. The paediatrician calls you for help as the delivered baby has respiratory distress. This neonate is later diagnosed with a congenital diaphragmatic hernia.

a) Name four other causes of respiratory distress in a newborn. 4 marks

Airway:

- Obstruction in the airway.
- Congenital anomalies including Pierre Robin syndrome.
- Macroglossia.
- Laryngeal or tracheal atresia.
- Subglottic stenosis.
- Vocal cord problems.
- Tracheo-oesophageal fistula.
- Tumours.

Pulmonary:

- Respiratory distress syndrome.
- Pneumothorax.
- Pleural effusion.
- Cysts, malformations.
- Hypoplasia.
- Emphysema.
- Surfactant deficiency.

Cardiovascular:

- Cyanotic and acyanotic defects.

- Arrhythmias.
- Cardiac failure.

Thoracic:

- Diaphragmatic hernia or paralysis.
- Pneumomediastinum.
- Chest wall deformities.

Neuromuscular:

- Central nervous injury.
- Encephalopathy.
- Infections.
- Seizure disorder.
- Myopathies.

Others:

- Sepsis.
- Hypoglycaemia.
- Acidosis.
- Hypothermia.
- Metabolic defects.
- Electrolyte problems.
- Anaemia.

b) What is the aetiology for a congenital diaphragmatic hernia? 2 marks

Dual hit hypothesis:

- Pulmonary hypoplasia is the primary disturbance, due to genetic and environmental factors. This then hampers the formation of the diaphragm.

- The consequent protrusion of abdominal contents into the thoracic cavity further hinders lung development — the second hit.

c) Name a few other conditions that are associated with a congenital diaphragmatic hernia. 2 marks

- Trisomy 13, 18 and 21.
- Fryns syndrome.
- Cornelia de Lange syndrome.
- Beckwith-Wiedemann syndrome.
- CHARGE syndrome.
- Structural abnormality — CVS, genitourinary, limb, CNS, palate.

d) Name any two factors of severity that worsen the outcome and increase mortality. 2 marks

- Absence of liver herniation — most reliable antenatal predictor of survival.
- Gestational age at diagnosis — most significant predictor of mortality.
- Near absence of diaphragm — poorer survival.
- Cardiac defects worsen outcome.
- A small contralateral lung or bilateral hernia is a poor prognostic sign.
- Others — severe pulmonary hypertension, low birth weight, low Apgar score at 5 minutes.

e) Based on embryology, what are the two types of congenital diaphragmatic hernia? 1 mark

- Bochdalek — 95% — failure of fusion of the pleuroperitoneal folds, posterolateral.
- Morgagni — 5% — a defect in the septum transversum, posterior to the sternum, retrosternal or parasternal.

f) What are the medical treatments for a congenital diaphragmatic hernia and how would you optimise the patient before the surgery? 5 marks

- Children with respiratory distress need resuscitation and medical stabilisation.
- Tracheal intubation and artificial ventilation immediately after delivery.
- Avoid mask ventilation to prevent gastric insufflation.
- Insertion of a nasogastric tube with continuous or intermittent suction to decompress the bowel.
- Early echocardiography to reveal cardiac defects, pulmonary hypertension and shunt.
- Pharmacological:
  - pulmonary vasodilators (nitric oxide); other agents — intravenous sildenafil or prostacyclin;
  - prostaglandin E1 (maintain patency of ductus arteriosus);
  - inotropes or vasopressors (to reduce shunt and improve organ perfusion);
  - neuromuscular agents (to aid ventilator synchrony).
- Aggressive ventilation — to induce hypocapnia and reduce pulmonary hypertension.
- Protective ventilation strategy, high-frequency oscillatory ventilation, ECMO.

g) This neonate mentioned above was taken to the operating theatre for emergency open surgery and repair after stabilisation; what are the intraoperative challenges in this neonate? 4 marks

- Need excellent communication amongst the whole team.
- A difficulty in ventilation, mainly the control of $PaCO_2$, which is worse with thoracoscopic repair.

- Keep circuit dead space to a minimum.
- End-tidal CO_2 traces are unreliable due to small tidal volumes (transcutaneous CO_2 monitoring can be helpful).
- Inhaled nitric oxide should be available if there is worsening pulmonary hypertension.
- Haemodynamic stability should be closely monitored.

References

1. Quinney M, Wellesley H. Anaesthetic management of patients with a congenital diaphragmatic hernia. *Br J Anaesth Education* 2018; 18(4): 95-101.

Q8 — Non-accidental injury

A 4-year-old girl is admitted to the accident and emergency department and the staff has raised the suspicion of a non-accidental injury.

a) What types of physical injury would raise concerns of abuse in a child of this age? 4 marks

- Head and/or abdominal trauma.
- Rib fractures.
- Slap marks.
- Eye injuries.
- Bite marks.
- Burns.
- Scalds.
- Bruises.

b) What timely action must be taken as a result of your concerns? 7 marks

- Concerns must be escalated to the appropriate named person in charge for child protection (often this is the lead paediatric anaesthetist/consultant paediatrician).
- Postoperative discussion with the parents and child by the consultant paediatrician and anaesthetist with or without the surgical team.
- If the concerns remain, then this documentation needs to be completed.
- All actions must be in the best interest of the child.
- Child safety and wellbeing must be ensured.
- Information shared with the concerned authorities — knowledge and consent of the patient and parents wherever possible.
- Any advice if needed must be sought from a Caldicott Guardian, defence organisation or the GMC.
- The hospital safeguarding/child protection team would be expected to make further appropriate investigations and involve child social care services, the courts or the police depending on the requirement.

c) List the parental factors that are known to increase the risk of child abuse. 5 mar

- Step parents.
- Parents with mental health issues.
- A history of parental abuse in childhood.
- Parents with substance abuse/misuse.
- Teenage parents.
- Disabled parents.

d) List the features of a child's past medical history that are known to increase the risk of child abuse. 2 mar

- Unplanned or unwanted children.
- Children with disabilities — physical, learning, illness-related.
- Children with behavioural problems.
- Prematurity.

e) List the modes of presentation in the case of child neglect. 2 mar

- Unkempt child.
- Underweight/failure to thrive.

References

1. Melarkode K, Wilkinson K. Child protection issues and the anaesthetist. *Br J Anaesth CEACCP* 2012; 12(3): 123-7.

Q9 — Epiglottitis

A 3-year-old child presents to the accident and emergency department with a short history of respiratory distress, fever, drooling and stridor.

a) List the differential diagnoses for this child's condition. 5 marks

Upper airway:

- Uvulitis.
- Epiglottitis.
- Croup.
- Retropharyngeal/peritonsillar abscess.

Lower airway:

- Tracheitis.
- Bronchiolitis.

Pulmonary:

- Pneumonia.
- Empyema.

b) What is the causative organism for epiglottitis? 1 mark

- The most common causative organism is *Haemophilus influenzae* type b (Hib).
- Other *Haemophilus* subgroups.
- *Streptococcus* species.

c) How would you initially manage this child? 6 marks

- History — onset, symptoms.
- Examination — this may need to be limited to avoid distressing the child.

Focus on:
- airway examination;
- respiratory rate, pattern, use of accessory muscles;
- the child's position — may assume a sniffing position;
- ability to swallow and drooling;
- if possible, assess circulatory status, conscious level, pupils, rash.

- Arrange for senior help (consultant anaesthetist, consultant ENT surgeon).
- Ensure that the parents are present and the child is comfortable.
- Avoid any invasive measures (cannulation) if the child becomes distressed/agitated.
- Antimicrobial therapy.
- Other measures — humified oxygen, steroids, nebulised adrenaline.
- Heliox, if available and tolerated by the child.
- Plan for definitive control of the airway and consider transferring to the operating theatre for airway management.

d) List the advantages of inhalational induction in this child. 4 mar

- A slow onset of anaesthesia and an ability to maintain a spontaneously breathing patient.
- If there is complete airway obstruction, no volatile agent will get to the patient and they will wake up.
- Less distressing as it does not require intravenous access prior to induction.
- Inhalational anaesthetics cause bronchodilatation.

e) List the potential advantages of intravenous induction in this child. 4 mar

- Rapid onset.
- A more commonly used technique by most anaesthetists so there is more familiarity with this technique.
- 100% oxygen can be provided.

- Even if the airway is not completely patent, anaesthesia can be maintained intravenously, thus avoiding awareness.

References

1. Davies I, Jenkins I. Paediatric airway infections. *Br J Anaesth Education* 2017; 17(10): 341-5.

Q10 — Palliative care in a child

A 6-year-old child is diagnosed to have severe spastic quadriplegic cerebral palsy. This boy is wheelchair-bound, has a gastrostomy, needs frequent suctioning due to excess secretions in the respiratory tract, and suffers with epileptic fits. In his recent intensive care admission, his respiratory failure is severe and his clinical condition deteriorates.

a) What are the priniciples of paediatric palliative care in general? 3 mar

- A holistic approach to life-limited children.
- Symptom management.
- Psychosocial management.
- Bereavement care.
- Highly complex, with a need to focus on multisystem needs, requires multidisciplinary involvement.
- Inter-disciplinary ethical decision-making, advance care planning.

b) Name a few standards of care in paediatric palliative care, based on the Together for Short Lives Core Care Pathway for children with life-limiting and life-threatening conditions. 6 mar

- Prognosis sharing and significant news — disclosure and provision of information.
- Transfer and liaison between hospital and community services.
- Multidisciplinary assessment of needs.
- Child and family care plan — ongoing, multi-agency care plan — health, social care and education sectors.
- End-of-life care plan — multi-agency care plan involving the child and family.
- Bereavement support plan — ongoing support, referral to specialist services.

c) What are the factors to consider in pain management in this child and what management strategies would you use? 4 marks

Factors:

- Cause of pain.
- Associated pathology.
- Psychosocial factors.
- Views of the patient and family.

Management:

- WHO pain ladder.
- Routes of administration of opioids.
- Neuropathic medications.
- Non-pharmacological approaches.

d) What are the factors to consider if this child has agitation and how would you manage it? 4 marks

Factors:

- Causes of agitation (pain, hypoxia, urinary retention, delirium, constipation).
- Psychological cause (anxiety or depression).
- Drug interaction possibility.

Management:

- Non-pharmacological strategies (calm quiet room, address fears and concerns).
- Benzodiazepines.
- Neuroleptic agents (haloperidol, levomepromazine).

e) If this child has nausea and vomiting, how would you manage this? 3 mark

- Education and prevention, reversible and associated causes, antiemetic medications, minimise strong odours, keep meals small and appetising.
- Medications — ondansetron (CTZ action), can be combined with steroids, cyclizine, levomepromazine, domperidone (caution, works at the vagal level), metoclopramide (caution, extrapyramidal effects), dexamethasone can lower ICP, haloperidol (CTZ and anxiolytic), chlorpromazine (CTZ), prochlorperazine (CTZ and vestibular centre).

References

1. Aidoo E, Rajapakse D. Overview of paediatric palliative care. *Br J Anaesth Education* 2019; 19(2): 60-4.

Q11 — Endoscopy in a child

An 8-year-old girl is listed for an upper and lower GI endoscopy on a gastroenterology list.

a) List a few conditions that would need endoscopy in a child of this age. 4 marks

- Inflammatory bowel disease.
- Functional GI disorders.
- Chronic intestinal pseudo-obstruction.
- Polyposis syndromes.
- Vascular disorders in the gut.
- Reflux oesophagitis, Barrett's oesophagus, oesophageal dysmotility.
- Achalasia.
- Varices.
- Gastric erosion, ulcers, gastritis, gastic outlet obstruction.
- Coeliac disease, peptic ulcer disease.
- Colitis, colonic dysmotility, polyps.
- Fissures, haemorrhoids.

b) How would you assess this child for anaesthetic need for the endoscopy? 3 marks

A full anaesthetic review and appropriate investigations should be conducted, with an emphasis on the following.

History:

- Nutrition.
- Reflux.
- Medications.
- Use of steroids.
- The need for antibiotic prophylaxis.

Examination:

- Bowel preparation can cause vomiting and diarrhoea, look for dehydration.

Investigations:

- Blood tests.
- Electrolyte disturbances to be checked.

c) Name a few anaesthetic techniques that could be used in this patient and describe how you would do them. 6 marks

- IV sedation — NICE recommends midazolam alone for OGD, and midazolam and fentanyl for colonoscopy (NICE CG 112, 2010).
- Laryngeal mask airway — i-gel® might be preferred, and a smaller than normal size might be needed.
- Spontaneous breathing without an adjunct — TIVA with propofol, oxygen via a nasal cannula, etCO_2 monitoring.
- Tracheal intubation — if less than 1 year or less than 10kg weight, difficult airway or airway problems, significant cardiac or respiratory comorbidity, increased risk of aspiration, specific procedures like PEG insertion.

d) What post-procedure care is needed after the endoscopy is done in this child? 3 marks

- Intraluminal gas might be left.
- Can cause diaphragmatic splinting, especially in small children.
- This can be worse if there is already respiratory or cardiovascular disease.
- Gentle pressure on the abdomen before extubation might help.
- Pain problems, especially with pre-existing abdominal pain.
- Rule out a bowel perforation if the pain is worse.

- Monitoring in recovery for residual effects of sedative drugs.
- Treat PONV if any.

e) List any four indications for tracheal intubation for endoscopic procedures in children. 4 marks

- Weight <10kg.
- Age <1 year.
- Aspiration risk.
- Difficult airway.
- Significant cardiac or respiratory comorbidity.
- History of obstructive sleep apnoea.
- Intense stimulating procedures such as PEG insertion.

References

1. Railton K, Lindley K, Wellesley H. Anaesthesia for children having endoscopy on a gastroenterology list. *Br J Anaesth Education* 2019; 19(3): 83-9.
2. Sedation in under 19s: using sedation for diagnostic and therapeutic procedures. NICE clinical guideline, CG112. London: National Institute for Health and Care Excellence, 2015. https://www.nice.org.uk/Guidance/CG112. Accessed on 11th July 2019.

Q12 — Pyloric stenosis

A 3-week-old preterm baby is admitted with complaints of projectile vomiting of non-bilious stomach contents and dehydration. A provisional diagnosis of hypertrophic obstructive pyloric stenosis is made by the paediatric team.

a) What is the aetiology of pyloric stenosis? 2 marks

- Hypertrophy of the smooth muscle of the pylorus, which forms the gastric outlet.
- Uncertain aetiology.
- Environmental and hereditary contributory factors are identified.
- A higher incidence in monozygotic than dizygotic twins. Genetic loci have been identified.
- The incidence is 0.9 to 5.1 per 1000 live births.
- 4-5 times higher in boys than girls.
- More common in first-born children.

b) What are the electrolyte changes that can occur in this patient and what is the mechanism for these changes? 6 marks

- Vomiting consists of gastric secretions, which are high in hydrogen and chloride ions, with some sodium and potassium, along with loss of water.
- Hypokalaemic hypocholoraemic metabolic alkalosis.
- Dehydration and a reduction in plasma volume.
- Aldosterone causes sodium and water retention, causing further potassium loss in urine (Na^+/K^+ exchange), worsening the hypokalaemia.
- Initially, bicarbonate is excreted in the urine to compensate for the alkalosis, leading to alkaline urine.
- Eventually, the kidneys excrete hydrogen to maintain plasma volume, resulting in a paradoxical acidic urine despite metabolic alkalosis.

- Medullary receptors cause ventilatory stimulation due to hydrogen ions.
- Increased $PaCO_2$, increased CSF hydrogen concentration.
- Metabolic alkalosis can cause respiratory depression and apnoea.
- Even if plasma pH is corrected, equilibration with CSF pH may take longer.

c) If the electrolyte changes are not corrected, can you take this patient to the operating theatre as an emergency to correct the stenosis? 2 marks

- Pyloric stenosis is a medical, not a surgical emergency.
- It is safer to wait for surgery while they are rehydrated and electrolyte abnormalities and alkalosis are corrected.

d) What are the surgical options in pyloric stenois? 2 marks

- Ramstedt approach — horizontal incision in the right upper quadrant, longitudinal incision through the pylorus muscle to the mucosa without perforating it.
- A curved circumumbilical skin incision is common now.
- Laparoscopic approach (increased risk of an inadequate myotomy, but there is less pain, and a shorter time to full feeds).

e) What are the anaesthetic considerations for this child with pyloric stenosis? 6 marks

- Risk of pulmonary aspiration of gastric secretions under GA.
- Need NG or orogastric tube insertion before induction (no need for constant suction before theatre as the electrolyte change can become worse).
- Check the depth and patency of the NG tube.
- Emptying the stomach might be done by rotating the infant from supine to lateral decubitus.

- Perform an ultrasound assessment of the gastric contents.
- Avoid hypoxaemia; complete neuromuscular block before intubation is vital.
- Ensure an adequate depth of anaesthesia before laryngoscopy.
- Use rapid-sequence intubation but avoid cricoid pressure as the infant airway is compressible and easily deformed.
- Remember that FRC is reduced, with greater oxygen consumption.

f) What are the analgesic techniques that you could use in this patient? 2 marks

- Ultrasound-guided rectus sheath block.
- TAP block.
- Local anaesthetic infiltration by the surgeon.

References

1. Craig R, Deeley A. Anaesthesia for pyloromyotomy. *Br J Anaesth Education* 2018; 18(6): 173-7.

Chapter 14

Pain

ANSWERS

Q1 — Persistent postoperative pain

a) Define persistent postoperative pain. 3 marks

Persistent postoperative pain is defined as pain having the following features:

- Pain that develops after a surgical procedure.
- Pain that is persistent for more than 2 months following a surgical procedure.
- Other causes for this pain have been excluded (e.g. infection, malignancy, etc).
- The possibility that pain is due to a pre-existing cause has been excluded.

b) List five surgical procedures that are most commonly associated with persistent postoperative pain. 5 marks

- Amputation.
- Thoracotomy.
- Cardiac surgery.
- Mastectomy.
- Breast augmentation.

- Iliac crease bone harvest site.
- Knee arthroplasty.
- Radical prostatectomy.
- Hernia repair.
- Caesarean section.
- Hip replacement.

c) What are the risk factors for the development of persistent postoperative pain? 8 mark

The risk factors are multifactorial.

Patient factors:

- Psychological factors such as catastrophisation, anxiety and depression can increase the risk.
- Preoperative pain in the operative area increases the risk of persistent postoperative pain.
- Inadequate and interrupted sleep increases the risk.
- Genetic differences/polymorphisms in pain processing, causing an altered sensitivity to pain, differences in opioid receptors and variations in metabolism of analgesics.
- Good descending noxious inhibitory control reduces the risk of persistent postoperative pain.
- The first 7 days median pain scores after a surgery are more predictive of persistent postoperative pain.
- Poor pain control with medications during the first week postoperatively due to factors like improper instructions to the patients for analgesia, patients fearing addiction to drugs such as opioids or patients experiencing analgesic-related adverse effects.
- Younger patients tend to have more persistent postoperative pain.

Surgical factors:

- There is more chronic persistent pain with open surgery compared with laproscopic surgery.
- Postoperative complications such as reoperation, infection, wound dehiscence, haematoma.
- Intraoperative non-identification of nerves causing damage due to diathermy or entrapment.

Anaesthetic factors:

- Regional anaesthesia including epidural anaesthesia (after amputations, thoracotomies, major intra-abdominal surgeries) or paravertebral blocks (for mastectomies) may be beneficial for reducing the incidence of persistent postoperative pain.
- Severe persistent acute post-surgical pain.
- The use of adjuvants in regional blocks, e.g. clonidine.

d) What pathophysiological changes occur at the spinal cord level during the transition from acute to persistent postoperative pain? 4 marks

- Central sensitisation — repetitive nociceptive stimuli, altered dorsal horn activity and amplification of sensory flow.
- Immune-mediated inflammatory reactions, hypersensitivity and ectopic neural activity.
- Expansion of receptive fields of central neurones.
- Reduced thresholds for responses at the spinal cord level.
- Activation of spinal cord microglial cells occurs which modulates the synaptic function.
- Altered expressions of Na^+ channels.

References

1. portal.e-lfh.org.uk — Pain (ePain).
2. Searle RD, Simpson KH. Chronic post-surgical pain. *Br J Anaesth CEACCP* 2010; 10(1): 12-4.

Q2 — Opioids, spinal cord stimulators and intrathecal pumps

a) How should you manage the perioperative opioid requirements of a patient who is having elective surgery and who takes regular opioids for non-malignant pain? 8 marks

A multidisciplinary team approach is required comprising patient education, planning for analgesia depending on the nature of surgery and implementing multimodal analgesia along with postoperative analgesic support — all key to optimising the outcomes:

- Early recognition of these complex patients by pre-assessment teams and surgeons followed by appropriate referrals to anaesthetists, pain specialists, psychologists, etc.
- Thorough patient assessment in terms of patient expectations, opioid doses and their side effects and the ability to engage with services like the pain team, physiotherapists, etc., as needed.
- Maximising the use of opioid-sparing techniques in the perioperative period — regular paracetamol, NSAIDs/COX2 inhibitors as appropriate along with local anaesthetic techniques ranging from local anaesthetic infiltration of the wound, the use of wound catheters for infiltration, regional anaesthesia or central neuraxial blockade.
- Other opioid-sparing medications like gabapentinoids, ketamine, clonidine and intravenous lignocaine infusions.
- Recognition and prevention of opioid withdrawal by continuing/replacing the preoperative opioids appropriately. Use conversion tables/equianalgesic doses to convert parent opioid to an oral or IV morphine equivalent dose to achieve this.
- Recognising that these patients are likely to need more opioids as compared with opioid-naïve patients and supplementing them with opioids in the form of IV PCA or orally as appropriate.

- Being mindful of opioid tolerance and opioid-induced hyperalgesia in this group of patients.
- Provide education on tapering strong opioids to the intended dose after discharge.

b) Give the conversion factors for oral tramadol, codeine and oxycodone to the equianalgesic oral morphine dose. 3 marks

- 67mg oral tramadol = 10mg oral morphine.
- 100mg oral codeine = 10mg oral morphine.
- 5mg oral oxycodone = 10mg oral morphine.

c) What are the perioperative implications of an existing spinal cord stimulator? 6 marks

Patients may present for surgery with an external (temporary) or internal (implanted) spinal cord stimulator.

For general and regional anaesthesia:

- Neuraxial blockade may be administered if essential, provided the site for the spinal/epidural needle or epidural catheter is away from the spinal cord stimulator implant and its wires. Fluoroscopic guidance is advisable if possible.
- Confirm the position/location of the spinal cord stimulator beforehand to know its location by operative records or radiological means.
- Electrocautery should be avoided if possible. If unavoidable, use a bipolar cautery rather than unipolar.
- If monopolar diathermy is unavoidable, then make sure that its earthing plate is kept as far away from the stimulator and its leads as possible.
- Consult with the device technician before and after surgery whenever possible.

- In peripheral nerve blocks, use an ultrasound-guided approach to localise the nerve rather than a peripheral nerve stimulator as it can interfere with the implant.
- The electrodes for defibrillation/cardioversion should be placed as much away from the leads and stimulator as possible. Use the lowest possible energy which is preferably done by a biphasic defibrillator.

d) What additional perioperative precautions should be taken if the patient has an intrathecal drug delivery system fitted? 3 marks

- Avoid spinal anaesthesia via a lumbar puncture route in the presence of intrathecal drug delivery (ITDD) systems.
- Avoid epidural anaesthesia at the level of the catheter insertion and connection. It may be administered above or below the level where the ITDD system is placed.
- Doses of IV opioids intraoperatively should be as for an opioid-naïve patient unless the patient is already on opioids via a route other than ITDD system opioids.
- ITDD pump malfunction is rare, but this will need appropriate technical support.
- In the case of a baclofen intrathecal pump, sudden malfunction of the pump can cause baclofen withdrawal, which is a medical emergency.
- Take appropriate precautions to minimise infections of ITDD systems.

References

1. Simpson GK, Jackson M. Perioperative management of opioid-tolerant patients. *Br J Anaesth Education* 2017; 17(4): 124-8.
2. Dose equivalent and changing opioids. Faculty of Pain Medicine, Royal College of Anaesthetists. https://www.rcoa.ac.uk/faculty-of-pain-medicine/opioids-aware/structured-approach-to-prescribing/dose-equivalents-and-changing-opioids. Accessed on 25th June 2019.

3. Whitney P-S, Sturgess J. Anaesthetic considerations for patients with neurosurgical implants. *Br J Anaesth Education* 2016; 16(7): 230-5.
4. Lynch L. Intrathecal drug delivery systems. *Br J Anaesth CEACCP* 2014; 14(1): 27-31.

Q3 — Neuropathic pain

a) What is neuropathic pain? 2 marks

Neuropathic pain is pain initiated or caused by a primary lesion or disease of the somatosensory nervous system.

b) List a few pain descriptors used by patients to describe their neuropathic pain. 2 marks

- Burning.
- Tingling.
- Electric shock-like.
- Radiating.
- Pins and needles.
- Stabbing.
- Shooting.
- Crawling sensation.
- Lancinating.
- Gnawing.
- Scalding.

c) List any four examples of neuropathic pain. 2 marks

- Trigeminal neuralgia.
- Post-herpetic neuralgia.
- Post-amputation pain.
- Painful diabetic neuropathy.
- Persistent post-surgical pain.
- Complex regional pain syndrome (CRPS).
- Central post-stroke pain.
- Post-spinal cord injury pain.

d) List any three commonly used medications to manage neuropathic pain and explain their mechanism of action. 6 marks

- Amitriptyline — tricyclic antidepressant.
- Gabapentin — alpha-2 delta ligand in calcium channel.
- Pregabalin — alpha-2 delta ligand in calcium channel.
- Duloxetine — SNRI (serotonin norepinephrine reuptake inhibitor).
- Tramadol — opioid and serotoninergic.
- Lignocaine patch — sodium channel blockade.
- Capsaicin cream or patch — TRPV1 activation.

e) What pain scales are used to assess neuropathic pain? 2 marks

- LEEDS Assessment of Neuropathic Symptoms and Signs (LANSS) scale.
- Douleur Neuropathique 4 (DN4) scale.
- Pain Detect scale.

f) Give examples of unidimensional pain scales. 3 marks

- Visual analogue pain scale.
- Verbal pain rating scale.
- Numerical pain rating scale.

g) Give examples of multidimensional pain scales. 2 marks

- Brief Pain Inventory (BPI).
- McGill Pain Questionnaire.

h) List any two pain assessment tools that you would use in a 5-year-old child after an appendicectomy in the immediate postoperative period. 1 mark

- Wong-Baker FACES® scale.
- Pieces of Hurt scale.
- Face, Legs, Activity, Cry, Consolability (FLACC) scale.

References

1 https://portal.e-lfh.org.uk/LearningContent/Launch/89833.

2. Bendinger T, Plunkett N. Measurement in pain medicine. *Br J Anaesth Education* 2016; 16(9): 310-5.

Q4 — Complex regional pain syndrome

A 37-year-old female is referred to the pain clinic with a possible diagnosis of complex regional pain syndrome (CRPS). She had a right wrist fracture and was in a plaster cast for 6 weeks. She developed severe pain even on light touch as soon as the cast was removed.

a) What is CRPS? 2 marks

Complex regional pain syndrome (CRPS) is a post-traumatic disorder consisting of a non-dermatomal distribution of continuous and severe pain in the affected limb, associated with varying combinations of sensory, motor, vasomotor, sudomotor, and trophic disturbances in the affected area.

b) How is CRPS classified? 1 mark

- CRPS type I — no demonstrable nerve lesion or damage.
- CRPS type II — nerve damage or lesion present.

c) List the symptoms and signs of CRPS from the Budapest diagnostic criteria and explain these criteria. 8 marks

Symptoms and signs from the Budapest criteria.

Symptoms (must report at least one symptom from three out of four categories):

- Sensory — suggestive of hyperalgesia and/or allodynia.
- Vasomotor — temperature asymmetry and/or skin colour changes and/or skin colour asymmetry.
- Sudomotor/oedema — oedema and/or sweating changes and/or sweating asymmetry.

- Motor/trophic — decreased range of motion and/or motor dysfunction (weakness, tremor, dystonia) and/or trophic changes (hair, nail, skin).

Signs (must have evidence of at least one sign from two out of four categories):

- Sensory — evidence of hyperalgesia (to pinprick) and/or allodynia (to light touch and/or deep somatic pressure and/or joint movement).
- Vasomotor — evidence of temperature asymmetry and/or skin colour changes and/or asymmetry.
- Sudomotor/oedema — evidence of oedema and/or sweating changes and/or sweating asymmetry.
- Motor/trophic — evidence of a decreased range of motion and/ or motor dysfunction (weakness, tremors, dystonia) and/or trophic changes (hair, nail, skin).

Other needed criteria:

- Continuing pain that is disproportionate to the initiating event.
- No other diagnosis can explain the signs and symptoms.

d) How would you manage and treat this patient with CRPS? 9 marks

- A multidisciplinary team approach, using a biopsychosocial model.
- Treatments can be classified into non-pharmacological, pharmacological and interventional.

Non-pharmacological:

- Early physical rehabilitation and early physiotherapy reduce pain and improve function.
- Psychologist input for patients with psychological issues such as an inability to cope or chronic pain behaviour.

- Laterality recognition, mirror-box therapy.
- Complimentary therapies like acupuncture and TENS have limited evidence.

Pharmacological:

- Medications for neuropathic pain — amitriptyline (tricyclic), gabapentin and pregabalin (alpha-2 delta calcium channel ligand), duloxetine (SNRI).
- Topical agents like lignocaine 5% plaster, capsaicin cream.
- N-acetyl cysteine intravenously.
- If vasomotor disturbance is prominent — calcium channel blockers, alpha-blockers or phosphodiesterase-5 inhibitors.
- If there is associated dystonia — give a muscle relaxant, e.g. baclofen.
- Intractable pain — low-dose IV ketamine, then converted to oral use.
- High-dose vitamin C — possible preventive role.
- Immunomodulators — glucocorticoids, anti-TNF-alpha, bisphosphonates.

Interventional:

- Sympathetic blocks; however, there is negative evidence published as per the updated EBGD (Evidence-based Guideline Development) guidelines for CRPS 1 (2014).
- Spinal cord stimulation — evidence-based — a positive effect on the somatosensory system and vasomotor disturbances.

References

1. Bharwani KD, Dirckx M, Huygen FJPM. Complex regional pain syndrome: diagnosis and treatment. *Br J Anaesth Education* 2017; 17(8): 262-8.

Q5 — Pain relief in cancer

You are asked to review a patient with advanced cancer on the medical ward for pain relief options.

a) List the causes of pain in a patient with advanced cancer. 5 marks

Cancer pain may be nociceptive, neuropathic or mixed (most common).

Causes can be:

- Cancer-related:
  - local mass effect on neural and non-neural tissues including bone inflammation, tissue invasion, ischaemia, compression, oedema;
  - paraneoplastic syndromes releasing anti-neuronal antibodies — leading to mononeuritis/polyneuritis and peripheral neuropathy.
- Cancer treatment-related:
  - chemotherapy-induced peripheral neuropathy;
  - radiation-induced neuropathic pain;
  - acute and chronic post-surgical pain.
- Associated condition-related:
  - immobilisation-related pain;
  - infection;
  - reactivation of *Herpes zoster* by immunosuppression.

b) How can side effects from opioid medications be minimised in these patients? 4 marks

- Use of non-opioids for analgesia, especially in the initial stages — opioid-sparing agents.
- Reduce the dose of opioids — start on a low dose for opioids and gradually titrate to build up the dose.
- Symptomatic management of side effects like pruritis and constipation.

- Opioid rotation — change of opioids considering their equianalgesic doses of other opioids. Always start at a half to two thirds of the calculated equianalgesic dose of opioids.
- Administration of specific antagonists, e.g. oral naloxone for opioid-induced constipation.

c) List the steps in the WHO analgesic ladder for cancer pain. 6 mar

Step 1:

- Non-opioids +/- adjuvants.
- Paracetamol.
- NSAIDs with adjuvants like gabapentinoids.
- Bisphosphonates.
- Steroids.
- Tricyclics.

Step 2:

- Weak opioids (codeine, dihydrocodeine and tramadol) + non-opioid +/- adjuvants.

Step 3:

- Strong opioids (morphine, oxycodone, fentanyl) + non-opioids +/- adjuvants.

d) What is the most commonly used class of drug used for the management of cancer pain and in what manner are they used to optimise their effect? 2 mar

Opioids are the most commonly used class of drugs for pain relief in cancer. Opioids are used for:

- 'Background' analgesia — provided by long-acting opioids.

- 'Break-through' pain management — achieved by intermittent doses of short-acting opioids.

e) Give three examples of interventional strategies, along with their indications, done by pain specialists to manage cancer pain. 3 marks

- Coeliac plexus block — for pancreatic cancer pain.
- Ganglion impar block — for anorectal pain arising from local malignancies, e.g. cancer of the rectum.
- Superior hypogastric plexus block — for pelvic cancer pain syndromes.

Other examples are:

- Peripheral nerve blocks, e.g. intercostal nerve blocks.
- Neurolytic procedures — peripheral and intrathecal.
- Intrathecal drug delivery (ITDD) systems.
- Percutaneous cervical cordotomy.

References

1. Scott-Warren J, Bhaskar A. Cancer pain management: Part I: General principles. *Br J Anaesth CEACCP* 2014; 14(6): 278-84.
2. Scott-Warren J, Bhaskar A. Cancer pain management: Part II: Interventional techniques. *Br J Anaesth CEACCP* 2015; 15(2): 68-72.

Q6 — Problems due to opioids

A 48-year-old male attends the pre-anaesthetic clinic with a chronic use of high-dose opioids for low back pain.

a) Enumerate the long-term side effects and concerns with opioids if used for non-cancer pain. 6 mark

- Nausea, vomiting, dizziness, dry mouth, sedation — usually patients become tolerant to these over a period of time.
- Prurutis — persists in long-term opioid intake.
- Constipation — persists in long-term intake of opioids.
- Respiratory depression.
- Hallucinations, drowsiness.
- Endocrine and hormonal dysfunction — influence on the hypothalamo-pituitary-adrenal axis and hypothalamo-pituitary gonadal axis to cause adrenal insufficiency and hypogonadism. This can cause reduced libido, amenorrhoea, erectile dysfunction, depression and fatigue.
- Immunological — immunomodulating effect leading to immune suppression.
- Opioid-induced hyperalgesia.
- Tolerance, physical dependence and addiction.

b) Define tolerance, physical dependence and addiction. 3 mark

- Tolerance — an increased dose of a drug is required to achieve the same effect.
- Physical dependence — if the drug is stopped or antagonised or its dose is reduced there is a withdrawal syndrome associated with it.
- Addiction — addiction is characterised by a behaviour that manifests as impaired control and compulsive use of a drug associated with its craving, despite the harm.

c) What is opioid-induced hyperalgesia (OIH)? 2 marks

Opioid-induced hyperalgesia is a state of nociceptive sensitisation caused, following the exposure to opioids. It is a paradoxical phenomenon wherein administration of an opioid can cause a pro-nociceptive state in the nervous system.

d) What are the presenting features of OIH? 2 marks

- Diffuse and widespread pain all over the body along with increased sensitivity.
- Pain does not respond to the administration of an increased dose of opioid.

e) How would you manage a patient with OIH? 2 marks

- Identification of OIH and differentiating from opioid tolerance and the progression of the underlying disease process.
- Slow and gradual reduction in the dose of opioids used for pain.
- The use of non-opioid strategies for pain management.

f) What would be your substitute drug with the aim of reducing opioids in this patient in a pain clinic? 2 marks

- Buprenorphine (sublingual).
- Methadone (orally).

g) What are the aims and principles of substitution therapy in such patients? 3 marks

- To reduce the associated harm from the use of a problem drug.
- To prevent a withdrawal reaction from the problem drug, thereby providing stability.
- To reduce preoccupation and craving associated with the problem drug.

References

1. https://portal.e-lfh.org.uk/LearningContent/Launch/98139.
2. Long-term harms of opioids. Faculty of Pain Medicine, Royal College of Anaesthetists. https://www.rcoa.ac.uk/node/21103. Accessed on 25th June 2019.

Q7 — Intrathecal opioids

a) What are the sites of action of intrathecal (IT) opioids? 2 marks

Intrathecal opioids bind to G-protein coupled receptors at presynaptic and postsynaptic areas in the lamina 1 and 2 of the dorsal horn of the spinal cord. The number of receptors are much higher in the presynaptic areas compared with the postsynaptic areas.

b) What are the intracellular and extracellular mechanisms of analgesic effect within the spinal cord following the administration of IT opioids? 6 marks

Complex mechanisms exist for the actions of intrathecal opioids.

At the presynaptic level:

- G-protein coupled receptor activation leads to potassium channel opening and calcium channel closure thereby reducing intracellular calcium.
- This causes a reduction of excitatory neurotransmitters (glutamate and substance P) from the C-fibres (presynaptic) thereby leading to reduced nociceptive transmission.

At the postsynaptic level:

- Opioids bind to postsynaptic receptors of the dorsal horn of the spinal cord causing potassium channel opening and activation of descending pathways causing analgesia.

Other theories of mechanism of actions include:

- Reduction of release of GABA and glycine (inhibitory neurotransmitters) from the dorsal horns in the inhibitory pathways leading to a reduction in nociceptive transmission.

- Increase in CSF adenosine activity. Adenosine causes hyperpolarisation through increased potassium transmission into the cells causing a reduction in the activity of neurones.

c) List the principal side effects of IT opioids. 4 mar

More common:

- Nausea and vomiting.
- Respiratory depression (most feared).
- Pruritis.

Others:

- Sweating.
- Sedation.
- Delayed gastric emptying.
- Urinary retention.

Note: intrathecal opioids have much lower side effects compared with other systemic administration routes.

d) List the factors that may increase the risk of postoperative respiratory depression following the administration of IT opioids. 5 mar

The risk of respiratory depression is increased by:

- A high dose of opioids.
- Low-dose lipophilic opioids — early respiratory depression (~1 hour).
- Low-dose hydrophilic opioids — late respiratory depression (up to 24 hours).
- Increasing age.

- Concomitant use of other sedatives.
- Co-administration of opioids in the first 24 hours after intrathecal administration.
- Positive pressure ventilation and coexisting respiratory disease such as COPD.

e) What is the role of antihistamines in opioid-induced pruritis? 2 marks

- There is no role for antihistaminics in pruritis if it is opioid-induced.
- The likely mechanism is through modulation of C-fibres centrally, which may be responsible for the itch response.

f) How would you manage opioid-induced pruritis? 1 mark

Naloxone low-dose continuous infusion at less than 2μg/kg/hr.

References

1. Hindle A. Intrathecal opioids in the management of acute postoperative pain. *Br J Anaesth CEACCP* 2008; 8(3): 81-5.

Q8 — Phantom limb pain

You are called to see a 74-year-old male patient who has had a below-knee amputation 24 hours ago. Despite using a patient-controlled analgesia (PCA) pump with intravenous morphine, he is still in severe pain.

a) Mention the possible causes/reasons for inadequate pain control in this patient. 4 marks

- Low dose of morphine in the PCA.
- Comorbidities leading to the administration of a reduced dose of analgesics — it is difficult to balance effective analgesia and increasing morbidity due to the side effects of polypharmacy.
- A combination of pains including stump pain (surgical wound pain — predominant element) and phantom pain.
- Extensive tissue trauma causing severe nociceptive pain.
- An associated neuropathic component of pain secondary to neural tissue injury.
- Pre-existing pain in the limb.
- Infection or haematoma in the stump.

b) How would you optimise perioperative pain control in a patient having an amputation of a lower limb? 6 marks

- Multimodal analgesia from the start of the procedure.
- Regional anaesthesia — either by epidural analgesia or a perineural catheter:
  - epidural analgesia (check coagulation status before). The appropriate timing of catheter insertion and removal with the anticoagulation protocols in patients having vascular insufficiency is important;
  - perineural catheter for a local anaesthetic infusion around the nerve (sciatic nerve +/- femoral nerve) placed by the surgeon

intraoperatively or by anaesthetists postoperatively. This is useful, especially in the first 72 hours postoperatively.

- Intravenous PCA, e.g. morphine, fentanyl, oxycodone, etc, if regional analgesia is inadequate or cannot be administered.
- Opioid-sparing drugs — paracetamol, NSAIDs (only if appropriate).
- For neuropathic pain — gabapentinoids (e.g. pregabalin 25-75mg per day to start with) or tricyclic antidepressants.
- Ketamine infusions in severe pain (0.1-0.2mg/kg/hour).

c) List the types of post-amputation pain that patients may present with. 3 marks

- Stump pain.
- Phantom limb pain.
- Mechanical pain (due to altered weight and force distribution).
- Back pain, especially in the rehabilitation phase.

d) List the features of post-amputation pain syndrome (phantom limb pain). 3 marks

- Pain is felt in the distal extremity of the amputated limb.
- Usually episodic pain that comes in short bouts lasting a few seconds to hours.
- Pain is described as burning, shooting or cramping in nature.
- Occurs in up to 80% of amputees.

e) Enumerate the pharmacological options available for managing post-amputation pain syndrome. 4 marks

Multimodal analgesia:

- Regional blockade — (preventive):
  - continous perineural blockade with local anaesthetic (e.g. ropivacaine 0.2%) solutions using elastometric or similar pumps,

postoperatively for the first few days in an attempt to reduce sensitization; there is some evidence to support this preventive approach;
  - perineural clonidine (alpha-2 agonist) as an adjuvant to the local anaesthetic infusion.
- Antineuropathic analgesic agents are the mainstay of management:
  - gabapentinoids — the use of pregabalin in a suitable dose to start with, e.g. 50mg BD followed by gradual uptitration as needed. Gabapentin — dose 100mg TDS to start with;
  - tricyclic antidepressants, e.g. amitriptyline or nortriptyline, if there are no contraindications;
  - ketamine — NMDA antagonist with antineuropathic, antinociceptive and antihyperalgesic properties;
  - memantine — NMDA antagonist with much less psychotropic effects (compared with ketamine);
  - salmon calcitonin subcutaneous injection — a neuropeptide with novel analgesic action, which has shown early promising results.
- Simple analgesics, including paracetamol, NSAIDs (if no contraindications), weak opioids — these can be tried and continued if found useful.

References

1. Neil MJE. Pain after amputation. *Br J Anaesth Education* 2016; 16(3): 107-12.

Q9 — Pain with fractured ribs

You are called to the emergency department to assess a 70-year-old man with known chronic obstructive pulmonary disease (COPD). He has sustained fractures to his 8th, 9th and 10th ribs due to a fall. He has no other injuries. He is currently on paracetamol and codeine which are not helping him with his pain relief.

a) List the possible respiratory effects of inadequate analgesia from fractured ribs. 3 marks

- Reduced rib movement with a consequent reduction in tidal volume — causes a predisposition to atelectasis due to hypoventilation.
- Impaired gas exchange — if there is a flail segment from fractured ribs, the underlying lung will be contused and oedematous. This can lead to intrapulmonary shunting and reduced oxygenation (PaO_2).
- A change in the mechanics of breathing.
- An inability to adequately clear out the chest secretions.

b) What are the secondary respiratory complications resulting from fractured ribs? 1 mark

- Pneumonia.
- Respiratory failure (with the need for respiratory support).

c) List the key management strategies in optimising the ventilation in a patient with fractured ribs. 4 marks

- Supplemental humidified oxygen.
- Adequate (multimodal) analgesia.
- Nebulised saline.
- Respiratory physiotherapy if the patient is able to cooperate.
- CPAP application if appropriate, e.g. flail segment.

- If respiratory failure ensues then sedation with mechanical ventilation will be needed.

d) What is the purpose of a rib fracture score? 2 mark

To risk stratify the patients so as to:

- Determine the level of care needed.
- Decide on the appropriate level of pain management.

e) How would you assess the adequacy of pain relief in this patient? 3 mark

- Direct questioning of the patient regarding analgesic adequacy.
- Assess the pain scores by using various pain scales like the numerical rating scale, visual analogue scale, etc.
- Physiologic parameters which may be indicative of an underlying pain issue such as heart rate, blood pressure, respiratory rate and depth.
- Check oxygen saturation (hypoxia may indicate inadequate chest wall movement due to pain).
- Ensure that the patient is able to deep breathe and cough well.
- Auscultation — to ensure good air entry bilaterally.

f) What are the measures used to manage analgesia following fractured ribs? 7 mark

- Simple analgesics — paracetamol, NSAIDs (if there are no contraindications), weak opioids.
- Strong opioids — IV morphine 0.1-0.2mg/kg titrated to effect followed by a slow-release preparation of morphine orally.
- IV patient-controlled analgesia (PCA) with a strong opioid, e.g. morphine — loading dose (up to 0.2mg/kg titrated) followed by bolus doses on PCA (1-2mg bolus to start with).

- The addition of opioid-sparing drugs such as gabapentinoids, e.g. pregabalin 25mg BD to start with.
- Regional analgesia:
  - epidural analgesia — the standard of care with higher rib fractures, multiple level fractures, a flail chest, respiratory compromise and in the presence of a chest drain, e.g. 0.25% levobupivacaine — a loading dose 5-10ml initially followed by an infusion of 0.1% levobupivacaine + fentanyl (2μg/ml) 5-15ml/hour;
  - paravertebral block with an infusion of local anaesthetic via a catheter in the paravertebral space, e.g. 0.25% levobupivacaine up to 30-40ml titrated to pain relief followed by an infusion of 0.1% levobupivacaine at 5-10ml/hour;
  - serratus plane block — to target thoracic intercostal nerves that lie deep to serratus anterior but also pierce the serratus muscle and come superficial to it. The superficial approach is preferred with local anaesthetic infiltration as a bolus followed by an infusion via a catheter;
  - other approaches such as intercostal blocks at multiple levels for multiple fractured ribs.
- Operative fixation — considered in patients with deteriorating pulmonary function or those with a flail chest or respiratory failure secondary to fractured ribs.

References

1. May L, Hillermann C, Patil S. Rib fracture management. *Br J Anaesth Education* 2016; 16(1): 26-32.

Q10 — Back pain

a) List the causes of mechanical (musculoskeletal) back pain. 3 marks

- Discogenic back pain.
- Facetogenic back pain.
- Back pain from the sacroiliac joints.

b) List five examples of red flags whilst assessing a patient for back pain. 5 marks

- Recent weight loss (unintentional/unexplained).
- Presentation <20 years and >50 years.
- History of significant trauma.
- History of cancer, steroid use, HIV infection or IV drug abuse.
- Cauda equina syndrome.
- Unwell systemically.
- Structural abnormality.

c) List three causes of nerve root pain. 3 marks

- Spinal stenosis.
- Disc herniation.
- Epidural adhesions.

d) What is the recommendation for paracetamol in managing mechanical back pain as per the NICE guidelines? 1 mark

Not to offer paracetamol as the only drug (single drug) for managing back pain.

e) What is the recommendation for opioids in chronic low back pain as per the NICE guidelines? 1 mark

Opioids should not be offered to manage chronic low back pain.

f) What is the role of epidural injections in low back pain as per the NICE guidelines? 2 marks

- Epidural injections with local anaesthetics and steroids should be used only in acute and severe sciatica.
- There is no role for epidural steroid injections in patients with neurogenic claudication with central canal stenosis.

g) When should you perform radiofrequency denervation of the median branch nerve in a case of chronic back pain? 1 mark

Radiofrequency denervation should be performed only after a positive response to the diagnostic median branch block.

h) List the non-invasive interventions for low back pain and sciatica. 4 marks

- Self-management of back pain — tailored advice about the nature of back pain to patients and encouragement to continue with their normal activities.
- Group exercise programme based on the patient's needs, capabilities and preferences.
- Psychological support — as part of a combined exercise programme.
- Manual therapy — only with an exercise programme with or without psychological therapy.

References

1. Jackson MA, Simpson KH. Chronic back pain. *Br J Anaesth CEACCP* 2006; 6(4): 152-5.
2. Low back pain and sciatica in over 16s: assessment and management. NICE guideline, NG59. London: National Institute for Health and Care Excellence, 2016. https://www.nice.org.uk/guidance/ng59/chapter/Recommendations. Accessed on 25th June 2019.

Q11 — Trigeminal neuralgia

a) List any five characteristic features of trigeminal neuralgia. 5 marks

- Unilateral facial pain.
- Pain in the distribution of one or more divisions of the trigeminal nerve.
- Stereotyped clinical features in the individual patient.
- Brief.
- Lancinating.
- Sharp pain.
- Shooting pain.
- Electric shock-like.
- Brought on by ordinary stimuli (eating, washing, shaving, cold air, etc.).

b) What are the pathophysiological causes of trigeminal neuralgia? 3 marks

- Hyper-excitable axons (secondary to injury).
- Central sensitisation.
- Demyelination of the trigeminal nerve root (secondary to vascular compression).

c) List any one cause of non-idiopathic secondary trigeminal neuralgia. 1 mark

- Cerebello-pontine angle tumour.
- Multiple sclerosis.

d) What investigations might help in the diagnosis of secondary trigeminal neuralgia? 1 mark

- MRI brain.
- Evoked potentials.
- Electrophysiological studies.

e) What is the first-line management for trigeminal neuralgia and give some examples? 3 marks

Pharmacological/conservative:

- Carbamazepine (first choice).
- Oxcarbazepine (better side effect profile).
- Other antineuropathic drugs.
- Phenytoin.
- Valproate.

f) What are the possible side effects with carbamazepine? 3 marks

- Drowsiness.
- Liver damage.
- Hyponatraemia.
- Ataxia.
- Toxic epidermal necrosis.
- Stevens-Johnson syndrome.

g) What are the interventional management options for trigeminal neuralgia? 4 marks

- Surgical microvascular decompression.
- Stereotactic radiation surgery of the trigeminal nerve (gamma knife).
- Percutaneous balloon compression.
- Percutaneous rhizolysis.
- RF ablation of the Gasserian ganglion.

References

1. Vasappa CK, Kapur S, Krovvidi H. Trigeminal neuralgia. *Br J Anaesth Education* 2016; 16(10): 353-56.
2. Van Kleef M, Van Genderen WE, Narouze S, *et al.* Trigeminal neuralgia. *Pain Practice* 2009; 9(4): 252-9.

Q12 — Post-herpetic neuralgia

A 57-year-old female had shingles 2 years ago in her right T8 dermatome and has suffered with severe pain in that dermatome since then. Her sleep and mood are significantly affected.

a) What is post-herpetic neuralgia? 1 mark

Chronic pain >3 months with skin changes in the distribution of one or more sensory roots after a *Herpes zoster* infection.

b) What is the cause of *Herpes zoster*? 2 mark

- Reactivation of the *Varicella zoster* virus (double-stranded DNA virus).
- The virus lies latent in the spinal and cranial sensory ganglion after chickenpox (*Varicella*) infection.
- About 20% develop neuralgia.

c) Describe the pathophysiology of pain in post-herpetic neuralgia. 4 mark

- Degeneration of the affected primary afferent neurones.
- Atrophy of the spinal dorsal horn, scarring of the dorsal root ganglion and loss of epidermal innervation.
- Spontaneous discharges in deafferented central neurones.
- Intrinsic changes in the CNS.
- High-frequency impulses in demyelinated α-β fibres.
- Sensitisation of intact C nociceptor fibres.
- Central sensitisation from sprouting of α-β fibres and loss of C-fibre input.
- There are three subgroups:
  - irritable nociceptors;
  - deafferentation with allodynia;
  - deafferentation without allodynia.

d) List any six risk factors for post-herpetic neuralgia. 3 marks

- Older age.
- Female.
- Severe acute pain.
- Severe rash within 3 days of onset.
- Prodrome of dermatomal pain before rash, especially with fever.
- Psychosocial predictors — anxiety, poor coping strategies.

e) How would you prevent post-herpetic neuralgia? 3 marks

- Primary chickenpox vaccine in childhood — less likely to experience latency and then reactivation.
- Zoster vaccine (live attenuated) — reduces neuralgia and the overall burden of illness.
- Antiviral medications — controls viral DNA replication, e.g. acyclovir, valaciclovir, famciclovir.
- The addition of oral steroids to acyclovir improves acute pain control, but does not prevent neuralgia.
- Amitriptyline started within 48 hours of the rash decreases prevalence, but there is limited evidence.

f) How would you treat post-herpetic neuralgia? 7 marks

- Multimodal treatment with a biopsychosocial approach; education of the patient is vital to reassure and engage in a pain management approach.
- Non-pharmacological — TENS, acupuncture.
- Anticonvulsants:
  - gabapentin, pregabalin — act at the alpha-2 delta subunit of presynaptic voltage-gated calcium channels on primary nociceptors;
  - NNT = 4;
  - NNH 4 for minor side effects and 12 for major side effects.

- Antidepressants:
  - tricyclics — two aromatic rings attached to the cycloheptane ring;
  - inhibits re-uptake of serotonin and norepinephrine;
  - amitriptyline, nortriptyline;
  - NNT = 2.64;
  - NNH = 5.6 for minor side effects and 17 for major side effects.
- Topical therapies:
  - topical lignocaine 5% plaster — blocks sodium channels;
  - capsaicin cream — vanilloid receptor agonist — acts on the TRPV1 receptor; depletes substance P from sensory nerve endings; NNT 3.2; NNH 4;
  - menthol — TRPM8 receptor.
- SNRI — duloxetine can be used as per neuropathic pain guidelines.
- Opioids should be avoided in chronic pain as there is no evidence of long-term efficacy.
- Other medications — ketamine (NMDA), clonidine (alpha-2 agonist) — are rarely used.
- Interventions:
  - local anaesthetic infiltration;
  - peripheral nerve blocks;
  - dorsal root ganglion blocks;
  - sympathetic nerve blocks;
  - epidural local +/- steroids;
  - paravertebral or erector spinae plane blocks.
- Others:
  - pscyhology;
  - pain management programmes.
- Invasive interventions, e.g. spinal cord stimulation.

References

1. Gupta R, Smith PF. Post-herpetic neuralgia. *Br J Anaesth Education* 2012; 12(4): 181-5.

Chapter 15

Cardiac anaesthesia
ANSWERS

Q1 — CABG complications

a) What are the central and peripheral neurological complications of coronary artery bypass surgery? 3 marks

- Stroke.
- Cognitive dysfunction.
- Visual field defects.
- Subtle sensory-motor deficits.

b) List any five risk factors for central neurological complications in these surgeries. 5 marks

Patient factors:

- Age >70 years.
- Significant cerebrovascular disease.
- Extensive aortic atherosclerosis.
- Diabetes mellitus.

Surgical factors:

- Open chamber surgical procedures.
- Duration of cardiopulmonary bypass >90 minutes.
- Perioperative haemodynamic instability.
- Multiple aortic manipulations (repeated clampings, cannulations).

CPB — equipment factors:

- Use of bubble oxygenators (rather than membrane oxygenators).
- Lack of arterial inflow line filters.
- Use of nitrous oxide.

c) What are the pathophysiologic mechanisms involved in the neurologic complications after these surgeries? 4 marks

- Hypoperfusion — poor cerebral autoregulation.
- Focal ischaemia:
  - emboli (air, atheroma, clots);
  - during open heart procedures;
  - from the aorta during cannulation/clamping;
  - intraventricular thrombi.
- Global ischaemia — severe hypoperfusion, circulatory arrest.
- Inadequate cerebral protection.
- Reperfusion injury.
- pH stat management — vasodilation could increase embolic load.

d) Name any four intraoperative techniques that are used for monitoring cerebral perfusion during cardiac surgery. 4 marks

- EEG — processed EEG such as BIS.
- Evoked potentials.
- Transcranial Doppler.
- Jugular oxymetry.
- Non-invasive optical spectroscopy.

e) List four techniques that could reduce the incidence of central neurological complications. 4 marks

- Avoidance of inadvertent hypotension.
- Reduce emboli during aortic cannulation — US scanning of aortic segment.
- Slow rewarming.
- Use of microfilters in the CPB circuitry.
- Meticulous de-airing techniques.
- Cerebral protection — pharmacological and non-pharmacological (cooling).
- Maintenance of euglycaemia.

References

1. Tan AMY, Amoako D. Postoperative cognitive dysfunction after cardiac surgery. *Br J Anaesth CEACCP* 2013; 13(6): 218-23.
2. Kaplan J. *Cardiac Anesthesia*, 7th ed. Philadelphia: Elsevier, 2016.

Q2 — Off-pump bypass

a) List four theoretical advantages of 'off-pump' coronary artery bypass (OPCAB) grafting compared with an 'on-bypass' technique. 4 marks

- Reduction in neurological complications.
- Less need for transfusion.
- Reduction in renal failure.
- Fast-track surgery.
- Cost benefits.
- Reduced postoperative temperature fluctuations and associated complications.

b) What are the four potential mechanisms of haemodynamic instability during OPCAB grafting? 4 marks

- Placement of stabilisers reduces contractility and thus stroke volume.
- Change in anatomical position of the heart chambers (e.g. verticalisation).
- Change in anatomical position of heart valves thus altering flow through the chambers.
- Reduced venous return.
- Ischaemia during the anastomosis.
- Arrhythmias.

c) List any three anaesthetic strategies that help to minimise this haemodynamic instability. 6 marks

- Careful assessment, selection and optimisation of patients.
- Close monitoring.
- Maintenance of coronary supply/demand balance.
- Maintenance of optimal core body temperature.

d) List three important mechanisms to maintain coronary perfusion during off-pump CABG. 3 marks

- Heart rate control (supply/demand balance).
- Maintain coronary perfusion with fluids (optimal preload) and vasopressors.
- Close communication with surgeons.
- Intracoronary (vessel) shunts.

e) What are the potential disadvantages of OPCAB grafting? 3 marks

- Potential for inadequate revascularisation.
- Inadequate data to compare with on-pump surgery on long-term results.
- Haemodynamic instability during surgical manipulation.

References

1. Alston RP, Myles PS, Ranucci M. *Oxford Textbook of Cardiothoracic Anaesthesia*. Oxford: Oxford University Press, 2015.
2. Kaplan J. *Cardiac Anesthesia*, 7th ed. Philadelphia: Elsevier, 2016.

Q3 — Cardiac tamponade

You are asked to review a 65-year-old woman on the cardiac intensive care unit who has undergone coronary artery bypass surgery earlier in the day.

a) List any six clinical features that might suggest the development of cardiac tamponade. 8 marks

- Sudden increase or decrease in drain output.
- Tachycardia.
- Hypotension.
- Reduced urine output.
- Dyspnoea.
- Decreased consciousness/disorientation.
- Muffled heart sounds.
- Pulsus paradoxus.

Beck's triad — hypotension, engorged neck veins and muffled heart sounds.

b) Name four investigations with their findings that could confirm the diagnosis of cardiac tamponade. 6 marks

- Reduced cardiac output.
- Raised CVP.
- ECG — electrical alternans.
- Echocardiogram — compression of heart chambers.
- CXR — enlarged heart.
- PA catheter — equalisation of pressures in heart chambers.

c) Outline the key steps of acute cardiac tamponade management in this patient. 4 marks

- Immediate sternotomy if in extremis.
- Induction in theatre.
- Surgeon scrubbed and ready.
- Blood available.
- Large-bore access.
- Careful induction — ketamine could be useful.
- Fluids and vasopressors to maintain coronary perfusion pressure.

d) Name any two other causes of cardiac tamponade. 2 marks

- Trauma.
- Iatrogenic damage during intracardiac pressure studies.
- CVP or PA catheter insertion procedures.
- Iatrogenic injury during coronary angiography and stenting.
- Heart chamber laceration during pericardiocentesis.

References

1. Alston RP, Myles PS, Ranucci M. *Oxford Textbook of Cardiothoracic Anaesthesia*. Oxford: Oxford University Press, 2015.
2. Kaplan J. *Cardiac Anesthesia*, 7th ed. Philadelphia: Elsevier, 2016.

Q4 — Implantable cardiac devices

a) List any four possible indications for the insertion of a cardiac implantable permanent pacemaker. 4 mar

- Sick sinus syndrome.
- Recurrent symptomatic bradycardia.
- Third-degree heart block.
- Advanced second-degree heart block.
- Heart rate less than 40.
- Ventricular pauses greater than 5 seconds.
- Periods of asystole more than 3 seconds.
- Trifascicular block.
- Biventricular pacing in patients with cardiac failure.

b) List any four possible indications for the insertion of a cardiac implantable cardioverter defibrillator (ICD). 4 mar

- VF/VT cardiac arrest.
- Symptomatic recurrent VT.
- Recurrent haemodynamically unstable SVT.
- Structural heart disease.
- Cardiomyopathy (ischaemic, dilated).
- Conduction disorders.
- Acquired or inherited spontaneous arrhythmogenic conditions.

c) What factors would you check/consider preoperatively in a patient with these types of devices? 6 mar

- History, examination and optimisation (of fluids, electrolytes and medications).
- Check device information — device type (pacemaker vs. ICD; pacemaker patient identification card).
- Time since last check of the device (6 months ICD; 12 months PPM).

- Battery life.
- ECG — to check the function and the patient's dependency on their pacemaker.
- CXR.
- Physiologist advice on the device.
- Determine the device behaviour with a magnet.
- Turn off advanced rate response function.
- The defibrillator function of an ICD should be deactivated immediately before any surgery where electromagnetic interference is deemed likely.

d) Outline the main features of intraoperative and postoperative management of patients with these types of devices having elective surgery under general anaesthetic. 6 marks

- Monitor ECG continuously.
- Consider invasive blood pressure monitoring to check mechanical capture (especially if poor ventricular function).
- Bipolar diathermy.
- If unipolar diathermy is used, minimise the effects.
- Defibrillation pads applied.
- Defibrillator pad placement to avoid/reduce electrical flow through intracardiac leads.
- Defibrillator capable of pacing readily available.
- Drugs for cardiopulmonary resuscitation immediately available.
- Stable induction and maintenance of anaesthesia.
- Consider avoiding succinylcholine.
- Back-up pacing and defibrillation facilities readily available in recovery.
- Postoperative device check and reprogramming if needed.
- Follow the ALS® algorithms to treat bradyarrhythmias and tachyarrhythmias.

References

1. Bryant HC, Roberts PR, Diprose P. Perioperative management of patients with cardiac implantable electronic devices. *Br J Anaesth Education* 2016; 16 (11): 388-96.
2. Kaplan J. *Cardiac Anesthesia*, 7th ed. Philadelphia: Elsevier, 2016.
3. Yao F-SF, Ed. *Yao & Artusio's Anesthesiology: Problem-Oriented Patient Management*, 8th ed. Philadelphia: Wolters Kluwer, 2016.

Q5 — One-lung ventilation

a) How can the risks associated with lung resection be quantified preoperatively? 6 marks

- ECG.
- CXR.
- ABG — PaO_2 <6kPa associated with poor oxygen saturation (<90%) is high risk; a drop in saturation with exercise by more than 4% is high risk.
- Pulmonary function tests (PFTs) — FEV1 <1.5L (for lobectomy) and <2L (for pulmonectomy) are high risk.
- Diffusion capacity — DLCO <80% is high risk; <60% increased mortality.
- Cardiopulmonary exercise testing (CPET) — <15ml/kg/min is high risk; <10ml/kg/min is associated with increased mortality.
- Quantitative lung scan (V/Q scan) — for predicted postoperative lung function (<40% is high risk).
- Simple CPET tests such as the 6-minute walk test (<400m needs further evaluation).
- Cardiac risk should be stratified.

b) List any six factors that can lead to the development of high airway pressures during one-lung ventilation (OLV). 4 marks

- Airway compression (internal or external).
- Secretions.
- Blood.
- Tissue soiling.
- Tube kinking.
- Malposition of the double-lumen tube (DLT) or migration of the blocker.
- Bronchospasm.
- Tension pneumothorax in the dependent (ventilated) side.
- Inadequate depth of anaesthesia and muscle relaxation.

c) How would you manage the development of hypoxaemia during OLV? 8 mar

- Confirm tube position (fibreoptic bronchoscopy).
- Increase FiO_2.
- Ensure haemodynamic stability — oxygen delivery.
- Optimise haemoglobin — oxygen delivery.
- CPAP of non-dependent lung.
- PEEP in dependent lung.
- Lung recruitment in the dependent (ventilated) side.
- Institution of two-lung ventilation.
- Jet ventilation.
- Clamping of the pulmonary artery on the operated side to reduce shunt.

d) What analgesic methods could be used for thoracic surgeries? 2 mar

- Epidural analgesia — PCEA.
- Paravertebral analgesia — single shot/continuous.
- Intercostal blocks.
- Wound infusions.
- PCA.

References

1. Gould G, Pearce A. Assessment of suitability for lung resection. *Br J Anaesth CEACCP* 2006; 6(3): 97-100.
2. Ng A, Swanevelder J. Hypoxaemia during one-lung anaesthesia. *Br J Anaesth* CEACCP 2010; 10(4): 117-22.

Q6 — Dilated cardiomyopathy

a) List any three presenting clinical features of dilated cardiomyopathy (DCM). 3 marks

- Palpitations (tachycardia).
- Breathlessness (dyspnoea).
- Fatigue.
- Pedal oedema.
- Ascites.
- TIA/stroke (emboli from LV thrombus).

b) What are the pharmacological and non-pharmacological management options for a patient with DCM? 5 marks

- ACE inhibitors.
- Loop diuretics.
- Beta-blockers.
- Spironolactone.
- Anticoagulants (LV thrombus).
- Biventricular (resynchronisation) pacing.
- Left ventricle assist devices.
- Heart transplantation.

c) List the predictors of poor outcome in patients with DCM undergoing surgery. 2 marks

- Left ventricular ejection fraction <20%.
- Elevated left ventricular end-diastolic pressure.
- Left ventricle hypokinesia.
- Non-sustained ventricular tachycardia.

d) What are the haemodynamic goals when anaesthetising patients with DCM? 4 mar

- Avoid tachycardia.
- Minimise cardiodepressant negative ionotropic (myocardial depression) effects of anaesthetic agents.
- Maintain preload.
- Prevent an increase in afterload (facilitates LV offloading).

e) What measures would you take to achieve these haemodynamic goals during anaesthesia? 6 mar

- Opioids have minimal myocardial depressant effects.
- Etomidate causes the least haemodynamic changes.
- Ketamine should be avoided (causes undesirable tachycardia and a rise in SVR).
- Careful titration of anaesthesia.
- Avoid sudden hypotension for maintaining organ perfusion.
- Invasive monitoring and guided fluid therapy.
- Maintain systemic vascular resistance with vasopressors.
- Maintain cardiac output (with inodilators such as phosphodiesterase inhibitors).
- Treat arrhythmias.
- Regional anaesthesia offers minimal haemodynamic changes.
- Central neuraxial blockade would increase forward cardiac output (by reducing afterload), but hypotension should be avoided.

References

1. Davies MR, Cousins J. Cardiomyopathy and anaesthesia. *Br J Anaesth CEACCP* 2009; 9(6): 189-93.
2. Ibrahim IR, Sharma V. Cardiomyopathy and anaesthesia. *Br J Anaesth Education* 2017; 17(11): 363-9.
3. Kaplan J. *Cardiac Anesthesia*, 7th ed. Philadelphia: Elsevier, 2016.

Q7 — Aortic stenosis surgery

A 70-year-old woman with aortic stenosis presents for an open aortic valve replacement (AVR).

a) What are the three most common aetiological causes of aortic stenosis? 3 mar

- Congenital (bicuspid valve).
- Rheumatic fever.
- Calcification (sclerosis).

b) What are the main pathophysiological factors responsible for deterioration in a patient with aortic stenosis? 4 mar

- Left ventricular outflow obstruction.
- Concentric LV hypertrophy.
- LV diastolic dysfunction.
- Myocardial ischaemia.
- Fixed stroke volume.
- LV failure.

c) Which specific symptoms may be used in assessing the progression of this woman's disease and correlate directly with 50% mortality? 3 mar

- Angina — 5 years.
- Syncope — 3 years.
- Dyspnoea (congestive heart failure) — 2 years.

d) Which specific cardiac investigations would you ask for in assessing this women preoperatively? 3 mar

- ECG — LV hypertrophy, arrhythmias (especially AF).

- Echocardiography — valve area, aortic root pathology, pathology in other valves, ventricular function.
- Angiography — coronary pathology, LV angiogram (function).

e) Give values for the peak aortic flow velocity, mean pressure gradient and valve area that would indicate that this woman has severe aortic stenosis. 3 marks

- Peak aortic flow velocity >4m/s.
- Mean pressure gradient >40mmHg.
- Valve area <1cm^2.

f) What would be your haemodynamic goals for the perioperative management of this patient? 4 marks

- Maintain myocardial oxygen delivery.
- Avoid tachycardia (adequate diastolic perfusion).
- Maintain contractility.
- Optimal preload.
- Treat arrhythmias and maintain sinus rhythm.

References

1. Chacko M, Weinberg L. Aortic valve stenosis: perioperative anaesthetic implications of surgical replacement and minimally invasive interventions. *Br J Anaesth CEACCP* 2012; 12(6): 295-301.
2. Alston RP, Myles PS, Ranucci M. *Oxford Textbook of Cardiothoracic Anaesthesia*. Oxford: Oxford University Press, 2015.
3. Kaplan J. *Cardiac Anesthesia*, 7th ed. Philadelphia: Elsevier, 2016.

Q8 — Lung resection and investigations

A 67-year-old male attends the clinic for a preoperative assessment before a right lower lobe lung resection for a localised non-small cell cancer.

a) Name any three bedside pulmonary function tests that could be done in this patient. 3 marks

- Ventilatory frequency.
- Cough strength and effectiveness.
- Pulse oximetry.
- Arterial blood gas.
- Lung volume measurements.

b) What are the diagnostic criteria for COPD based on spirometry? 1 mark

Global initiative for chronic Obstructive Lung Disease (GOLD):

- Post-bronchodilator FEV1/FVC <70% is a key criterion for diagnosis.
- May be overdiagnosed in the elderly; the ratio is important if it is less than the lower limit of normal (LLN) for that patient.

c) What does lung carbon monoxide transfer factor (TLCO) indicate and what is its significance? 2 marks

- TLCO indicates parenchymal lung function.
- It is severely impaired in interstitial lung disease and fibrosis.
- TLCO is also reduced in emphysema (reduced surface area for gas exchange).

d) What suggestive values of FVC (forced vital capacity) might need mechanical ventilation in neuromuscular diseases? 2 marks

- FVC of <20ml/kg.
- 30% decrease in FVC or maximal inspiratory or expiratory pressures.

e) What is the NICE guidance on preoperative testing with regards to spirometry in the normal general population? 1 mark

NICE does NOT recommend routine preoperative spirometry for any groups of patients.

f) In the above question with regards to the patient's lung resection, what is the role of pulmonary function tests (PFTs) and how would you interpret them? 6 marks

- The aim of PFTs is to identify patients with a high risk of cardiorespiratory morbidity and mortality.
- To assess the magnitude of risk.
- Tests for respiratory mechanics:
  - FEV1 is a good indicator of pulmonary reserve;
  - FEV1 <60% can have significant postoperative complications;
  - FEV1 <30% can increase risks by 60%.
- Tests for lung parenchymal function:
  - TLCO and % predicted postoperative TLCO;
  - both are prognostic of long-term survival after surgery.
- Test for cardiopulmonary reserve:
  - stair climbing test;
  - shuttle walk test;
  - CPET studies;
  - VO_2 max less than 15ml/kg/min — increased morbidity;
  - VO_2 max less than 10ml/kg/min — increased mortality.

g) Name a few techniques of calculating the ppo (predicted postoperative) pulmonary function. 3 marks

- Anatomical calculation.
- Ventilation/perfusion scintigraphy.
- Quantitative CT scanning.
- Dynamic perfusion MRI.

h) What are the selection criteria for the suitability of lung volume reduction surgery (LVRS)? 2 mark

NICE guidelines:

- FEV1 and TLCO both more than 20% predicted.
- $PaCO_2$ less than 7.3kPa.
- Upper lobe predominant emphysema on high-resolution CT.

References

1. Ntima NO, Lumb AB. Pulmonary function tests in anaesthetic practice. *Br J Anaesth Education* 2019; 19(7): 206-11.
2. Routine preoperative tests for elective surgery. NICE guideline, NG45. London: National Institute for Health and Care Excellence, 2016. https://www.nice.org.uk/guidance/ng45. Accessed on 1st July 2019.

Q9 — Cardiac transplantation in children

A 13-year-old child is listed in the cardiac theatre for a heart transplantation for end-stage heart failure.

a) What are the indications for cardiac transplantation in children? 2 marks

- Dilated cardiomyopathy (idiopathic or associated with metabolic, neuromuscular, infection, viral and genetic disorders, and drugs) — the most common indication for a cardiac transplant in children.
- Hypertrophic cardiomyopathy, restrictive cardiomyopathy (rare), non-compaction cardiomyopathy.
- Congenital heart disease — single or biventricular system.
- Retransplantation.

(International Registry of Paediatric Heart and Lung Transplantation — ISHLT.)

b) Name four factors that are important in organ allocation with regards to transplantation. 4 marks

- ABO blood compatibility.
- Size matching (donor-recipient weight ratio — DRWR) (between 0.7 to 2 is better).
- Sex-matched transplants.
- Human leukocyte antigen (HLA) matching; panel reactive antibody (PRA) test.

c) What factors would you consider during induction of anaesthesia in this child? 2 marks

- Patients receiving mechanical support — ventricular assist device (pulsatile or centrifugal type) — to be continued.

- If there is no support, this is a high risk and very cautious induction is needed.
- Cardiac surgeons and perfusion team to be ready if needed.

d) How would you manage intraoperatively? 2 mark

- Anticipate and prepare for difficult central venous access.
- Prepare for haemodynamic instability during reperfusion.
- Prepare for haemorrhage and instability.
- Prepare to support the transplanted heart mechanically and pharmacologically.

e) What immunosuppressant therapies are you aware of for induction therapy and maintenance therapy? 2 mark

- Induction — antithymocyte antigen is the preferred agent in children; others include Interleukin-2 antagonist (basiliximab) or high-dose methylprednisolone.
- Maintenance — a combination of a calcineurin inhibitor (tacrolimus) and cell cycle inhibitor (mycophenolate mofetil) and a short-term course of oral steroids (prednisolone).

f) What are the complications that can occur after transplantation? 4 mark

- Primary graft failure — low cardiac output syndrome in the early hours or days post-transplant.
- Rejection — acute cellular rejection (ACR) in the first 6 months post-transplant, T-cell mediated, or antibody-mediated rejection (AMR) which presents later, humoral-mediated.
- Cardiac allograft vasculopathy — a leading cause of death in the medium- to long-term.
- Infection — CMV, EBV, bacterial.
- Malignancy — post-transplant lymphoproliferative disease (PTLD).

g) If this child has a successful transplant and presents to you for an elective surgery at a later date, what factors would you consider? 4 marks

- Elective — discussion with the transplant centre if appropriate.
- Emergency — urgent consult with the transplant centre; echocardiography locally before discussion.
- Find out if the child is compliant with immunosuppressant therapy.
- Clinical status of the child.
- Reasonable differential diagnosis.
- Due to immunosuppressive drugs, there can be fewer obvious signs of infection or impaired renal function — be aware.

References

1. Black CS, Khushnood A, Holtby H, Hepburn L. Cardiac transplantation in children. *Br J Anaesth Education* 2019; 19(4): 105-12.

Q10 — Right ventricular failure

A 69-year-old obese female presents with a significant history of obstructive sleep apnoea with presenting features of right ventricular failure. She has been using a CPAP machine for the last 4 years.

a) What are the signs of acute right ventricular failure? 2 marks

- Signs due to a low cardiac output.
- Signs due to systemic venous congestion.
- Signs of hypoperfusion — deranged liver function, raised urea, creatinine and lactate.
- Decreased venous oxygen saturation.

b) What are the signs of chronic right ventricular failure? 2 marks

- Ascites.
- Exertional dyspnoea.
- Reduced exercise tolerance.
- Ankle swelling.

c) Describe one investigation that will help in the early diagnosis for right ventricular failure. 1 mark

Transthoracic echocardiogram (TTE).

d) Discuss the pathophysiology of right ventricular failure. 4 marks

- Volume or pressure overload or reduced contractility.
- Dysfunction triggered by injury or stress.
- Acute — MI, pulmonary embolism.
- Chronic — pulmonary hypertension, congenital cardiac disease.
- Multiple compensatory mechanisms — hypertrophy, extracellular matrix expansion, reduction in wall stress, upregulation of neurohormonal systems.

- Increased preload — tricuspid regurgitation, atrial septal defects.
- Increased afterload — pulmonary hypertension, pulmonary embolism.
- Decreased contractility — RV infarction, arrhythmias, sepsis.

e) How can obesity lead to right ventricular dysfunction? 2 marks

- Obesity — an independent risk factor for cardiovascular disease.
- Increased cardiac output.
- Obesity-hypoventilation syndrome.
- Obstructive sleep apnoea.
- RV dilatation, increased RV wall thickness seen in young obese patients.

f) What is the mechanism of right ventricular failure in obstructive sleep apnoea? 2 marks

- Apnoeic episodes leading to hypoxic pulmonary vasoconstriction.
- Remodelling of pulmonary microcirculation results.
- Increased pulmonary vascular resistance, pulmonary hypertension, RV dysfunction.
- Negative intrathoracic pressure, increased venous return, increased preload in the RV.
- Coexisting cardiovascular disease and hypoxaemia.

g) List the management strategies for a patient admitted with right ventricular failure. 7 marks

- Identify the cause and treat it.
- Optimise heart rate:
  - higher rate;
  - aim for sinus rhythm.
- Optimise rhythm:
  - cardioversion if there are new-onset rhythm problems;
  - amiodarone +/- cardioversion.

- Optimise preload:
  - filling;
  - small fluid boluses 50ml with CVP monitoring;
  - if overfilled, loop diuretics;
  - haemofiltration if needed.
- Augment contractility and maintain perfusion:
  - inodilators — dobutamine, milrinone;
  - vasopressors — noradrenaline.
- Minimise afterload:
  - prevent hypoxia, acidosis, hypercapnia;
  - reduce PEEP;
  - inhaled or IV pulmonary vasodilators.
- Surgical management — mechanical circulatory support:
  - balloon pump;
  - ECMO;
  - ventricular assist devices.

References

1. Murphy E, Shelley B. Clinical presentation and management of right ventricular dysfunction. *Br J Anaesth Education* 2019; 19(6): 183-90.

Chapter 16

Intensive care
ANSWERS

Q1 — Major haemorrhage

A 45-year-old man has a major haemorrhage following significant trauma and is admitted to the emergency department. He does not have a head injury.

a) Give any two definitions of a major haemorrhage. 2 marks

- Loss of more than one blood volume within 24 hours (approximately 70ml/kg).
- 50% of total blood volume lost in less than 3 hours.
- Bleeding in excess of 150ml/minute.
- Bleeding leading to a systolic blood pressure of <90mmHg and a pulse of >110 bpm.

b) What are the principles of management of a major haemorrhage in this patient? 8 marks

- Ensure that the appropriate team members are contacted (activate the trauma team).
- Activation of the major haemorrhage protocol.
- Identification of the source of bleeding.
- Control/prevention of further blood loss.

- High-flow oxygen/airway control.
- Establish IV or IO access.
- Baseline bloods.
- Frequent measurement of Hb and coagulation using point-of-care tests (such as TEG®/ROTEM®/HemoCue®/ABG to guide transfusion).
- Frequent measurement and correction of electrolyte abnormalities.
- Transfusion of blood and coagulation products to restore organ perfusion.
- Measures to maintain/achieve normothermia.
- Consider imaging and/or damage control surgery.
- Consider the use of antifibrinolytics (e.g. tranexamic acid).

c) List any three metabolic complications that might follow a massive blood transfusion. 3 marks

- Hypothermia.
- Acid base abnormalities (metabolic alkalosis, acidosis).
- Electrolyte abnormalities — hypocalcaemia, hyperkalaemia/ hypokalaemia, hypomagnesaemia.
- Citrate toxicity.

d) What are the immunologic complications that can occur after a massive blood transfusion? 3 marks

- Transfusion-related lung injury (TRALI).
- Transfusion-associated immunomodulation (TRIM).
- Transfusion related graft-vs-host disease.

e) What are the other complications that might follow a massive blood transfusion? 4 marks

Transfusion reactions:

- Immediate haemolytic transfusion reactions and non-haemolytic febrile reactions.

- Allergic reactions.

Others:

- Coagulopathy.
- Transfusion-related infections.
- Transfusion-associated circulatory overload (TACO).

References

1. Gaunt C, Woolley T. Management of haemorrhage in major trauma. *Br J Anaesth CEACCP* 2014; 14(6): 251-5.
2. Maxwell MJ, Wilson MJA. Complications of blood transfusion. *Br J Anaesth CEACCP* 2006; 6(6): 225-9.
3. ATLS®: Student course manual, 10th ed.

Q2 — Nutritional support in intensive care

A 45-year-old man with a history of ulcerative colitis and alcohol abuse is admitted to the intensive care unit for inotropic and ventilatory support following a laparotomy to excise a toxic megacolon. His Body Mass Index is 18kg/m^2.

a) Why should this patient receive early nutritional support? 3 marks

- Critically ill patient — major surgery, multi-organ failure, sepsis.
- Critical illness is associated with an increased energy requirement and catabolism.
- There is a high risk of malnutrition and refeeding syndrome — low BMI, alcohol abuse.

b) List any four clinical benefits of early nutrition. 4 marks

- Better wound healing.
- Prevention of loss of muscle mass.
- Decreased ventilator dependence.
- Decreased ICU length of stay.
- Improved immune function.

c) What are the routes of nutrition and daily energy requirements for this patient? 2 marks

- The enteral route of nutrition is preferred as the initial choice.
- A parenteral route can be used if the enteral route is not tolerated.
- Energy target — 25kcal/kg/day.
- Increase to target over 2-3 days.

d) What are the basic nutritional requirements in critical illness? 6 marks

Table 16.1

Carbohydrate	2g/kg/day
Protein	0.8-1.2g/kg/ day
Fat	1g/kg/day
Water	30ml/kg/ day
Sodium, chloride	1-2mmol/kg/day
Potassium	0.8-1.2mmol/kg/day
Calcium, magnesium	0.1mmol/kg/day
Phosphate	0.2-0.5mmol/kg/day

e) List two advantages of enteral nutrition. 2 marks

- Cheaper and easier mode.
- Lower risk of infection.
- Preservation of integrity of the gut mucosa.

f) List three disadvantages of enteral nutrition. 3 marks

- Increased association with ventilator-associated pneumonia.
- Requires intact gut function.
- Less reliable delivery of energy.
- Risk of displacement of nasogastric tubes.
- Risk of aspiration.
- Feed intolerance, diarrhoea.

References

1. Nutrition support for adults: oral nutrition support, enteral tube feeding and parenteral nutrition. NICE clinical guideline, CG32. London: National Institute for Health and Care Excellence, 2017. https://www.nice.org.uk/Guidance/CG32. Accessed on 1st July 2019.
2. Chowdhury R, Lobaz S. Nutrition in critical care. *Br J Anaesth Education* 2019; 19(3): 90-5.

Q3 — Ventilator-associated pneumonia

a) What are the key features in the definition of ventilator-associated pneumonia (VAP)? 3 marks

- Pneumonia occurring more than 48 hours after endotracheal intubation and mechanical ventilation.
- The presence of new or progressive chest infiltrates.
- Signs of systemic infection (fever, altered WBC count).
- Changes in sputum characteristics.
- Detection of a causative agent.

b) List the risk factors for the development of VAP. 8 marks

- Mechanical ventilation more than 48 hours' duration.
- Elevation of gastric pH.
- Large volume aspiration.
- Use of nasogastric tubes.
- Prolonged sedation and paralysis.
- Supine position.
- Use of TPN.
- Prior antibiotic therapy.
- Severe illness (APACHE score >18).
- ARDS.
- Coma.
- Burns.
- Recent abdominal/thoracic surgery.
- Multi-organ failure.
- Malnutrition.
- Alcoholism.
- Immunocompromised status.
- Malignancy.
- Diabetes mellitus.
- Azotemia.
- Acidosis.

c) What measures could be taken to reduce the risk of development of VAP? 8 marks

Non-pharmacologic:

- Alcohol-based hand washing policy.
- Elevation of the head of the bed (30-45°).
- Daily sedation interruption and assessment of readiness to extubate.
- Non-invasive ventilation.
- Heat moisture exchanger use.
- Use of silver-coated antimicrobial ETTs.
- Use of ETTs with a subglottic suction drainage port.
- Appropriate ETT cuff pressure control.
- Oral rather than nasal intubation.
- Use of closed suction catheters and sterile suction catheters.
- Avoidance of scheduled ventilator circuit changes.
- Kinetic beds.

Pharmacologic:

- Selective digestive decontamination.
- Avoid CNS depressants.
- Stress ulcer prophylaxis with sucralfate (controversial).

Methods to improve host immunity:

- Maintain nutritional status.
- Early discontinuation of invasive devices if possible.
- Treat disease states that affect host defences.
- Avoid agents that impair pulmonary defences (aminophylline, corticosteroids, sedatives).

d) What are bundles of care? 1 mark

- Grouped evidence-based practices (to encourage consistent practices).

References

1. Gunasekera P, Gratrix A. Ventilator-associated pneumonia. *Br J Anaesth Education* 2016; 16(6): 198-202.
2. Cairo JM. *Pillbeam's Mechanical Ventilation – Physiological and Clinical Applications*, 6th ed. Missouri: Elsevier, 2015.

Q4 — Acute respiratory distress syndrome

a) List the criteria for a diagnosis of acute respiratory distress syndrome (ARDS). 3 marks

- Timing — within 1 week of a known clinical insult or new/worsening respiratory symptoms.
- Chest imaging (CXR or CT) — bilateral opacities not fully explained by effusions/lung collapse.
- Origin of oedema — respiratory failure not fully explained by cardiac failure or fluid overload (objective assessment [echocardiography] is needed if there is no risk factor present).

b) How would you classify ARDS? 3 marks

ARDS is diagnosed according to the Berlin definition and is characterised as mild, moderate and severe depending on the paO_2/FiO_2 ratio:

- Mild — paO_2/FiO_2 26.6kPa to ≤39.9kPa with PEEP or CPAP ≥5cm H_2O.
- Moderate — paO_2/FiO_2 13.3kPa to ≤26.6kPa with PEEP or CPAP ≥5cm H_2O.
- Severe — paO_2/FiO_2 ≤13.3kPa with PEEP ≥5cm H_2O.

c) List any four clinical indices to quantify oxygenation in ARDS. 4 marks

- Partial pressure of arterial oxygen (paO_2).
- Fraction of inspired oxygen (FiO_2).
- PaO_2/FiO_2 ratio.
- Oxygen saturation (SpO_2).
- Oxygenation index — lower is better.
- Alveolar partial pressure of oxygen.
- Alveolar — arterial oxygen tension gradient.

d) What are the ventilatory strategies in managing a patient with ARDS? 5 marks

- Lung protective ventilation (6ml/kg of IBW tidal volume; plateau pressure ≤30cm H_2O [ARDSnet protocol]).
- Optimal PEEP.
- Prone ventilation.
- Lung recruitment manoeuvres.
- Inverse ratio ventilation.
- High-frequency oscillation ventilation (HFOV).
- Extracorporeal membrane oxygenation (ECMO).
- Weaning protocols with spontaneous breathing trials (when ready to wean).

e) What are the non-ventilatory strategies in managing a patient with ARDS? 5 marks

- Conservative fluid management.
- Neuromuscular blockade in the early phase of severe ARDS.
- Steroids (not recommended for routine use).
- Ensure adequate nutrition.
- Prevent complications of critical illness.
- Stress ulcer prophylaxis.
- VTE prophylaxis.
- Glucose control.
- Statins, inhaled NO, ketoconazole — the existing evidence does not support these therapies.

References

1. McCormack V, Tolhurst-Cleaver S. Acute respiratory distress syndrome. *Br J Anaesth Education* 2017; 17(5): 161-5.
2. Cairo JM. *Pillbeam's Mechanical Ventilation – Physiological and Clinical Applications*, 6th ed. Missouri: Elsevier, 2015.

Q5 — Sepsis, qSOFA and sepsis bundles

a) Define sepsis and septic shock. 2 marks

- Sepsis — life-threatening organ dysfunction caused by a dysregulated host response to infection.
- Septic shock — a subset of sepsis in which the underlying circulatory and cellular/metabolic abnormalities are profound enough to substantially increase mortality.

b) What are the features of RED FLAG sepsis? 8 marks

- Responds only to voice or pain or unresponsive.
- Acute confusional state.
- Systolic BP <90mmHg or drop >40mmHg from normal.
- Heart rate >130 per minute.
- Respiratory rate ≥25 per minute.
- Needing oxygen to keep SpO_2 ≥92%.
- Non-blanching rash, mottled/ashen/cyanotic.
- Anuric in the last 18 hours.
- Urine output less than 0.5ml/kg/hr.
- Lactate ≥2mmol/L.
- Recent chemotherapy.

c) What are the criteria of the qSOFA (quick SOFA) score? 3 marks

- Respiratory rate ≥22/min.
- Altered mentation.
- Systolic blood pressure ≤100mmHg.

d) How is the qSOFA score useful? 2 marks

- Quick, rapid bedside assessment.
- Prompts further investigations for organ dysfunction.

- Useful to initiate/escalate care as appropriate.
- Prompts to increase the frequency of monitoring or referral to critical care.
- A qSOFA score ≥2 predicts increased mortality.

e) List the elements of sepsis bundle interventions. 5 mar

- Measure lactate level (repeat if initial lactate >2mmol/L).
- Obtain blood cultures before the administration of antibiotics.
- Administer broad-spectrum antibiotics.
- Begin rapid administration of 30ml/kg crystalloid for hypotension or lactate ≥4mmol/L.
- Apply vasopressors if hypotensive or after fluid resuscitation to maintain MAP ≥65mm Hg.

An hour-1 bundle is a group of interventions, all of which should begin in the first hour from sepsis recognition but may not be necessarily completed within the first hour.

References

1. Singer M, Deutschman CS, Seymour CW, *et al*. The third international consensus definitions for sepsis and septic shock (Sepsis-3). *JAMA* 2016; 315(8): 801-10.
2. The UK Sepsis Trust; https://sepsistrust.org.
3. Levy MM, Evans LE, Rhodes A. The Surviving Sepsis Campaign bundle: 2018 update. *Critical Care Medicine* 2018; 46(6): 997-1000.

Q6 — Transfer of critically ill patients

You are asked to transfer a 43-year-old male patient from an intensive care unit to a specialised neurointensive care unit in a hospital 1 hour away by ambulance.

a) What are the technical risks with regards to the transfer of patients from critical care units? 3 marks

- Need a high level of care.
- Appropriately stabilised and resuscitated before transfer.
- Requires physical movement.
- Restricts positioning, monitoring, intervention and examination.
- Ventilation, BP maintenance and heart rhythm maintenance could be problematic.
- Unreliable power for equipment for monitoring, infusion pumps and ventilation.
- Unreliable oxygen supply.
- Venous access problems during transfer and mobilisation.
- Problems with transfer equipment.

b) What are the non-technical risks that are to be noted during the transfer of critical care patients? 3 marks

- Non-availability of adequate staff for the transfer compared with intensive care units.
- Work in isolation during transfer.
- Teams might be unfamiliar with each other and the patient.
- Issues with communication and liaison with different critical care units.

c) Describe the organisational risks in the transfer of critically ill patients. 2 mar

- Need to be aware of guidelines from the Association of Anaesthetists of Great Britain & Ireland (AAGBI), Royal College of Anaesthetists (RCoA) and Intensive Care Society (ICS).
- The hospital should have a designated consultant for transfers and audit/training.
- Standardisation of protocols, equipment and documentation.
- More burden on the preparing staff and the remaining staff.
- Must not jeopardise the remaining patients.
- Accompanying staff to be safely returned to base after transfer.
- A dedicated transfer service is ideal.

d) What guidelines are you aware of regarding the transfer of critically ill patients? 2 mar

- AAGBI guidelines 2009, 2006.
- ICS guidelines, 2011.
- NICE guidelines NG94, July 2017.
- Scottish Intercollegiate Guidelines Network, SIGN 139, May 2014.

e) What would you consider in the process of transfer? 2 mar

- Who? — the decision to transfer should be agreed with senior responsible consultants and team.
- With whom? — trained personnel, teamwork.
- When? — well prepared transfer, striking a balance between speed and safety.
- How? — appropriate and careful preparation, guidelines to be followed and a pre-departure checklist to be used.
- With what? — drugs, equipment, mode of transport.

f) Describe the essentialities in an ABCDE approach with regard to the transfer of a sick patient. 5 marks

- A — secure tracheal tubes, check and record before the transfer.
- B — adequate ventilation, saturation probes, $etCO_2$ monitoring, release pneumothorax, calculate oxygen needs, bag valve masks in need.
- C — appropriate resuscitation, two IV access sites secured well, arterial and other lines secured, vasopressors calculated, specialist equipment if needed.
- D — sedation/analgesia/paralysis, pumps for infusions, seizures to be well controlled.
- E — immobilisation of trauma patients as appropriate, all drains and tubes fixed securely, avoid hypothermia and monitor.
- Packaging — take care to avoid heat loss and injury, and avoid pressure areas.
- Documentation — every 5 minutes for vital signs, standardised across networks, duplicates for audit and incident reporting.

g) List the communication processes that are essential in the transfer of sick patients. 3 marks

- Firstly, referring and receiving senior consultants should discuss the transfer.
- The referring unit should document a care summary and handover letter.
- The transfer team should receive a handover in detail.
- The transfer team should hand over the patient clearly to medical and nursing staff, with details of any change during the transfer.

References

1. Bourn S, Bourn S, Wijesingha S, Nordmann G. Transfer of the critically ill adult patient. *Br J Anaesth* Education 2018; 18(3): 63-8.

Q7 — Propofol-related infusion syndrome

a) What is propofol-related infusion syndrome (PRIS)? 3 marks

- PRIS was first described in the paediatric population but increasingly it is seen in adult intensive care patients.
- A rare and fatal condition.
- Seen in children and also adults receiving a high dose (>5mg/kg/hr) of a propofol infusion and/or for more than 48 hours.
- Defined as acute refractory bradycardia leading to asystolic cardiac arrest in patients receiving a propofol infusion and in the presence of one or more of following:
  - metabolic acidosis — base deficit ≥10mmol/L;
  - rhabdomyolysis or myoglobinuria;
  - plasma lipaemia;
  - hepatomegaly/fatty liver.

b) What are the clinical effects of PRIS? 4 marks

- Metabolic acidosis — as a result of renal failure and increased lactate production.
- Cardiac changes — initial arrhythmias such as atrial fibrillation, supraventricular tachycardias, bundle branch blocks, bradycardias and eventually asystole.
- Lipidaemia — lipid metabolism is impaired due to increased sympathetic stimulation, high circulating cortisol and growth hormone levels. There is also a blockade of mitochondrial fatty acid oxidation.
- Rhabdomyolysis — from necrosis of skeletal and cardiac muscle. Leads to increased serum creatine kinase levels and myoglobinuria.
- Hepatomegaly, elevated liver enzymes.
- Acute kidney injury.

c) List the risk factors for PRIS. 5 mar

- Major head injuries.
- Sepsis.
- High exogenous/endogenous catecholamine and glucocorticoid levels.
- Low carbohydrate to high lipid intake.
- Inborn errors of fatty acid oxidation.

d) What specific laboratory findings might be expected in a case of PRIS? 3 mar

- Hyperkalaemia.
- Lipidaemia.
- Elevated liver enzymes.
- Raised lactate.
- Acute kidney injury (elevated serum creatinine).

e) How may PRIS be prevented? 3 mar

- Avoid using propofol doses of >5mg/kg/hr for more than 48 hours.
- Use other sedative agents in combination with propofol.
- Monitor serum creatine kinase, lactate and pH if using prolonged infusions.

f) How would you manage PRIS? 2 mar

- Discontinue the propofol infusion.
- Cardiovascular support with inotropes/vasopressors.
- Renal replacement therapy.
- Management of metabolic/electrolyte abnormalities.
- ECMO.

References

1. Loh N-HW, Nair P. Propofol infusion syndrome. *Br J Anaesth CEACCP* 2013; 13(6): 200-2.

Q8 — Guillain-Barré syndrome

A 68-year-old man is referred to the neurointensive care unit with suspected Guillain-Barré syndrome.

a) What is Guillain-Barré syndrome (GBS) and what are its causes? 5 mar

Guillain-Barré syndrome (GBS) is:

- An acute demyelinating polyneuropathy.
- An autoimmune response following a gastrointestinal or respiratory tract infection.
- Characterised by areflexia, motor weakness and CSF abnormalities.

Causes of GBS:

- Gastrointestinal or respiratory infection with pathogens such as *Campylobacter jejuni*, Epstein-Barr virus, *Mycoplasma pneumoniae* and *Cytomegalovirus*.
- As a complication of HIV infection.
- Other associations such as vaccines, surgery, epidural anaesthesia, bone marrow and organ transplant, SLE, lymphoma, sarcoidosis.

b) List the clinical features of GBS. 5 mar

- Motor weakness, progressive and usually ascending.
- Areflexia.
- Bulbar weakness and facial palsy.
- Ophthalmoplegia.
- Severe pain.
- Sensory involvement and symptoms.
- Respiratory muscle weakness leading to respiratory failure.
- Autonomic dysfunction leading to arrhythmias, labile blood pressure, fluctuations in heart rate, urinary retention, increased sweating and ileus.

c) List the investigations/findings that can be used to aid the diagnosis. 6 marks

- Routine blood tests — FBC, urea and electrolytes, liver function tests, renal function tests, clotting screen, calcium, inflammatory markers.
- Antibody tests to detect antiganglioside antibodies which are associated with a poorer prognosis. It is possible to also detect antibodies to the causative organism.
- Blood cultures.
- Stool cultures — to detect a *Campylobacter* infection.
- ECG — may show evidence of arrhythmias, ST depression, T wave inversion and a prolonged QT interval.
- CT of the head — to exclude raised intracranial pressure before performing a lumbar puncture.
- Lumbar puncture and CSF analysis — typically, increased protein and cells $<10/mm^2$.
- Electrophysiological studies — to aid the diagnosis and help differentiate from other conditions such as critical illness polyneuropathy.
- Gadolinium-enhanced spinal MRI.

d) What supportive treatment is needed in this patient with GBS? 2 marks

- Counselling.
- Nutritional support and dietetic input.
- Analgesia.
- Thromboembolic prophylaxis.
- Respiratory support.
- Physiotherapy and occupational therapy.

e) What specific therapies are available for GBS? 2 marks

- Intravenous immunoglobulins.
- Plasma exchange.

- Corticosteroids.
- CSF filtration.

References

1. Richards KJC, Cohen AT. Guillain-Barré syndrome. *Br J Anaesth CEPD Reviews* 2003; 3(2): 46-9.

Q9 — Renal replacement therapy

a) What are the renal indications for starting renal replacement therapy (RRT) in the intensive care setting (ICU)? 4 marks

- Rapid increase in serum urea and creatinine.
- Uraemic encephalopathy.
- Hyperkalaemia resistant to medical treatment.
- Severe metabolic acidosis.
- Oliguria or anuria.

b) What are the non-renal indications for starting RRT in the ICU? 4 marks

- Fluid overload.
- Toxin clearance.
- Severe electrolyte abnormalities.
- Temperature regulation.
- In severe sepsis, to remove inflammatory mediators.

c) List the types of RRT available in intensive care. 6 marks

- Intermittent haemodialysis (IHD).
- Continuous renal replacement therapy (CRRT):
  - continuous veno-venous haemofiltration (CVVH);
  - continuous veno-venous haemodialysis (CVVHD);
  - continuous veno-venous haemodiafiltration (CVVHDF);
  - slow continuous ultrafiltration (SCUF);
  - hybrid therapies (IHD and CRRT).

d) Outline the principal mechanisms of solute and water removal by filtration. 3 marks

- Convective process.
- Similar to the physiological filtration process in a nephron.

- Hydrostatic pressure gradients filter plasma, water and solute across a membrane.
- Works on the principle of a 'solute drag' — solute particles are dragged along with the mass movement of solvent across a membrane.
- Dependent upon direction and magnitude of transmembrane pressure.

e) Outline the principles of haemodialysis. 3 mark

- The underlying principle is diffusion across a membrane.
- Dialysate is pumped in a counter-current fashion to the blood flow.
- Diffusion across a membrane occurs as per the concentration gradient.
- This leads to a rapid equilibration of solutes.

References

1. Gemmell L, Docking R, Black E. Renal replacement therapy in critical care. *Br J Anaesth Education* 2017; 17(3): 88-93.
2. Standards and recommendations for the provision of renal replacement therapy on intensive care units in the United Kingdom. Intensive Care Society Standards and Safety, 2009.

Q10 — Refeeding syndrome

a) What is the daily energy requirement of a normal healthy 70kg man? 1 mark

25-35kcal/kg/day (NICE recommendations).

b) What are the recommended daily proportions of carbohydrate, fat and protein? 3 marks

- Carbohydrates — 50%.
- Fats — 35%.
- Proteins — 0.8-1.5g protein/kg/day (or 0.13-0.24g nitrogen/kg/day).

c) What is refeeding syndrome? 2 marks

A sudden carbohydrate load after a little or no nutritional intake for >/=5 days causing severe electrolyte abnormalities (due to the intracellular movement of phosphates, fluids and electrolytes).

d) What are the three major electrolyte abnormalities seen in refeeding syndrome? 3 marks

- Hypophosphataemia.
- Hypokalaemia.
- Hypomagnesaemia.

e) What is the commonest electrolyte nutritional deficiency? 1 mark

Hypophosphataemia.

f) Which patients are at particular risk of refeeding syndrome? 6 mark

- Patients who abuse alcohol.
- Chronically undernourished patients.
- Patients on diuretics.
- Patients on chemotherapy.
- Patients on insulin.
- Patients on antacids.
- Critically ill patients with no or minimal intake for >5 days.

g) How should the nutritional requirements of those 'at risk' be managed? 4 marks

- Identify the patients at risk of refeeding syndrome.
- For the first 2 days, commence nutritional support at 50% of estimated energy requirements in this at-risk group of patients.
- Increase by 200-400kcal every day thereafter.
- Electrolytes and micronutrients to accompany nutrition and fluids.
- Close monitoring and correction of serum electrolytes — potassium, magnesium, phosphate after feeding is started.

References

1. Macdonald K, Page K, Brown L, Bryden D. Parenteral nutrition in critical care. *Br J Anaesth CEACCP* 2013; 13(1): 1-5.
2. Nutrition support for adults: oral nutrition support, enteral tube feeding and parenteral nutrition. NICE clinical guideline, CG32. London: National Institute for Health and Care Excellence, 2017. https://www.nice.org.uk/Guidance/CG32. Accessed on 1st July 2019.

Q11 — Intra-abdominal hypertension

A 52-year-old male is admitted to the intensive care unit with a provisional diagnosis of intra-abdominal hypertension and oliguria.

a) Define intra-abdominal hypertension (IAH) and abdominal compartment syndrome. 2 marks

- Intra-abdominal hypertension — sustained abdominal pressure above 12mmHg.
- Abdominal compartment syndrome — sustained intra-abdominal pressure >20mmHg associated with organ dysfunction/failure.

b) Name any four causes of IAH. 4 marks

- Blunt or penetrating abdominal trauma.
- Haemorrhage — AAA rupture.
- Intestinal obstruction.
- Pregnancy.
- Ascites.
- Ileus.
- Burns.
- Intra-abdominal sepsis.
- Cirrhosis.
- Obesity.
- Intra-abdominal malignancy.

c) What are the pathophysiological consequences of abdominal compartment syndrome? 4 marks

- Cardiac — decreased venous return and increased SVR leading to decreased cardiac output and hypotension.
- Pulmonary — decreased thoracic volumes, a decrease in the P/F ratio and hypercarbia.

- Renal — decreased GFR and low urine output.
- Abdominal viscera — decreased perfusion.
- Neurologic symptoms can include increased ICP and a decrease in cerebral perfusion pressure (CPP).

d) How would you grade the severity of the IAH? 4 marks

- Grade I — intra-abdominal pressure 12-15mmHg.
- Grade II — intra-abdominal pressure 16-20mmHg.
- Grade III — intra-abdominal pressure 21-25mmHg.
- Grade IV — intra-abdominal pressure >25mmHg.

(World Society of the Abdominal Compartment Syndrome classification.)

e) What techniques could be used to measure intra-abdominal pressure? 2 marks

Direct method:

- Using pressure transducers (needle or intraperitoneal catheters).

Indirect method:

- Intravesicular catheter pressures (e.g. Foley catheter).

f) How would you manage the IAH in this patient? 4 marks

Non-invasive:

- NG tube placement for gastric decompression.
- Rectal tube placement for colonic decompression.
- Neuromuscular blockade to decrease abdominal compartment pressures in the ventilated ICU patient.

Invasive:

- Percutaneous drainage of abscesses, ascites or fluid from the abdominal compartment.
- Surgical decompression.

The prevention and early treatment of the potential cause may prevent the progression of IAH to abdominal compartment syndrome.

References

1. Berry N, Fletcher S. Abdominal compartment syndrome. *Br J Anaesth CEACCP* 2012; 12(3): 110-7.
2. Cripps MW, Perumean JC. Abdominal compartment syndrome. *BMJ Best Practice Topics* 2018, Mar 19.

Q12 — Stroke and thrombolysis

a) What imaging modalities are recommended by NICE in acute stroke? 2 marks

- Non-contrast CT scan.
- CT angiogram.
- Diffusion-weighted MRI, MR angiography.
- Carotid angiogram.

b) What specific treatments can be considered for acute thrombotic ischaemic strokes? 3 marks

Non-surgical treatment:

- Aspirin.
- Thrombolysis with alteplase within 4.5 hours of symptom onset.
- Intra-arterial thrombolysis and thrombectomy.
- Full-dose anticoagulation with heparin and later warfarin — acute venous stroke.

Surgical treatment:

- Decompressive hemicraniectomy.

c) What are the other general and supportive treatment measures that you would implement in the treatment of an acute stroke? 3 marks

- Supplemental oxygen if the SpO_2 is below 95%.
- Maintain blood glucose between 4-11mmol/L.
- Control of BP.
- Adequate nutrition and hydration.

- Early mobilisation.
- Prevent aspiration pneumonia.

d) In these patients, what is the potential consequence of severe hypertension? 1 mark

Severe hypertension causes haemorrhagic transformation and cerebral oedema.

e) What level of hypertension (systolic and diastolic) is regarded as severe after an ischaemic stroke? 2 marks

Severe hypertension after a stroke >220/110mmHg.

f) What is the recommendation for arterial BP values in patients for thrombolysis? 1 mark

Arterial BP should be lowered below 185/110mmHg.

g) A patient has had a large hemispheric infarction following a stroke. Outline your management of this patient following admission to critical care. 8 marks

- Nurse at 30° head up.
- Ventilation:
  - intubate if there are signs of respiratory insufficiency or neurological deterioration;
  - aim for normocapnia ($PaCO_2$ 4.5-5.0kPa).
- Sedation:
  - the use of barbiturates is discouraged;
  - sedation holds should be guided by ICP monitoring and clinical condition;
  - blanket daily wake-up trials are not recommended.

- Thrombolysis:
  - still of benefit in this population if commenced within 4.5 hours;
  - the impact on future plans for surgical decompression should be considered.
- Arterial pressure control:
  - MAP should be maintained >85mmHg;
  - systolic BP should be maintained at less than 220mmHg.
- Nutrition — SALT assessments are mandated before oral feeding is recommenced.
- Glycaemic control — maintain blood glucose at 7.8-10mmol/L.
- A transfusion threshold of 70g/L is recommended.
- DVT prophylaxis:
  - use intermittent pneumatic compression rather than stockings;
  - prophylactic LMWH;
  - early mobilisation for haemodynamically stable patients.
- Osmotherapy for cerebral oedema — mannitol and hypertonic saline.
- Prophylactic antibiotics, steroids and seizure prophylaxis are not recommended.

References

1. Redgrave J, Ellis H, Eapen G. Interventional therapies in stroke management: anaesthetic and critical care implications. *Br J Anaesth Education* 2017; 17(2): 43-7.
2. Stroke and transient ischaemic attack in over 16s: diagnosis and initial management guidance. NICE guideline, NG128. London: National Institute for Health and Care Excellence, 2019. https://www.nice.org.uk/guidance/ng128/chapter/Recommendations. Accessed on 1st July 2019.

Q13 — Diabetic ketoacidosis

You are asked to review an 18-year-old male in the emergency department who has been found obtunded at home. He is an insulin-dependent diabetic with a history of poor control. Capillary blood glucose is 23.4mmol/L.

a) List the biochemical findings that confirm the diagnosis of diabetic ketoacidosis (DKA). 2 marks

The diagnostic triad of DKA is:

- Ketonaemia ≥3.0mmol/L or significant ketonuria (more than 2+ on urine sticks).
- Blood glucose >11.0mmol/L or known diabetes mellitus.
- Bicarbonate <15.0mmol/L, venous pH <7.3, or both.

b) What are the clinical features of DKA? List at least two signs and two symptoms. 2 marks

Symptoms:

- Thirst, polyuria, polydipsia.
- Nausea, vomiting.
- Abdominal pain.
- Lethargy.
- Could even be the first presentation of DM.

Signs:

- Dehydration.
- Tachycardia, hypotension.
- Kussmaul respiration.
- Ketotic breathing.
- Altered consciousness, confusion.

c) What other clinical and biochemical findings are seen in severe DKA? 2 mark

The presence of one or more of the following:

- GCS less than 12 or abnormal AVPU scale.
- Oxygen saturation below 92% on air assuming normal baseline respiratory function.
- Systolic BP below 90mmHg.
- Pulse over 100 or below 60 bpm.
- Blood ketones over 6mmol/L.
- Bicarbonate level below 5mmol/L.
- Venous/arterial pH below 7.0.
- Hypokalaemia on admission (under 3.5mmol/L).
- Anion gap above 16 (anion gap = $[Na^+ + K^+] - [Cl^- + HCO_3^-]$).

These patients should be referred to the ICU/HDU.

d) What is the pathophysiology of DKA? 1 mark

- Relative or absolute insulin deficiency.
- Increase in counter-regulatory hormones.
- Hyperglycaemia due to gluconeogenesis, glycogenolysis, and impaired glucose utilisation by peripheral tissues.
- Free fatty acid release and their oxidation in the liver to ketones.
- Hydrogen ions produced by the dissociation of the ketone bodies cause metabolic acidosis.
- Hyperglycaemia causes an osmotic fluid shift from intracellular to extracellular compartments.
- Hyperglycaemia causes osmotic diuresis and loss of sodium, potassium, phosphate, water and glucose.

e) What are the three most common causes of DKA? 3 marks

- An underlying infection.
- Missed insulin treatment.
- First presentation of diabetes mellitus.

f) What investigations would you request in such a presentation of DKA? 3 marks

Mandatory investigations:

- Capillary ketone levels/urinalysis for ketones.
- Blood sugar.
- Blood gas for pH, bicarbonate, or both.

Routine investigations:

- Full blood count.
- Urea.
- Creatinine.
- Potassium.
- Sodium.
- Chloride.
- CRP.
- Liver function tests.

Investigations to detect the cause:

- ECG.
- Cultures.
- Amylase.
- Pregnancy test.

Ongoing investigations:

- Hourly CBG/arterial blood glucose and capillary blood ketones.
- 2-hourly pH, bicarbonate and potassium.

g) Outline the management plan for severe DKA within the first hour. 4 marks

- Resuscitation — ABCDE approach.
- Intravenous fluid — normal saline.
- Fixed rate IV insulin infusion at 0.1 units/kg/hour.
- Establish appropriate monitoring and investigations.
- If systolic BP <90mmHg, then administer a 500ml normal saline infusion over 15 minutes. Repeat if the patient remains hypotensive. Refer to intensive care if haemodynamic instability continues.
- Treatment of hyperkalaemia or hypokalaemia.
- If the patient takes a long-acting insulin, continue this at the normal dose and normal time.

h) What are the serious complications that can follow the management of DKA? 1 mark

- Cerebral oedema.
- Hypoglycaemia.
- Hypokalaemia, hyperkalaemia.
- Pulmonary oedema.

i) What is the mechanism of hypokalaemia in DKA and how is it managed? 2 marks

Potassium loss is caused by:

- A shift of potassium from the intracellular to extracellular space in exchange for hydrogen ions which accumulate in acidosis.

- A loss of extracellular potassium through osmotic diuresis.

Management:

- No potassium should be added to the initial litre of fluid.
- Subsequent fluids should have 40mmol/L of potassium chloride, provided the serum potassium is <5.5mmol/L, and the patient is not oliguric.

References

1. Hallett A, Modi A, Levy N. Developments in the management of diabetic ketoacidosis in adults: implications for anaesthetists. *Br J Anaesth Education* 2016; 16(1): 8-14.
2. Dhatariya K, Savage M, *et al*. Joint British Diabetes Societies Inpatient Care Group. The management of diabetic ketoacidosis in adults, 2nd ed., 2013. http://www.diabetes.org.uk/Documents/About%20Us/What%20we%20say/Management-of-DKA-241013.pdf. Accessed on 1st July 2019.

Q14 — Scoring systems, NEWS and ICNARC

Scoring systems are routinely used in intensive care units for critically ill patients.

a) What is a scoring system? 1 mark

- Scoring systems integrate easily measured data from patients into a statistical algorithm to provide a single score.
- This helps to predict the progress of a patient's illness and how they will respond to a clinical intervention.

b) What types of scoring systems are you aware of in critical care patients? 2 marks

- Illness severity scores — Sequential Organ Failure Assessment (SOFA).
- Outcome prediction models — Acute Physiology and Chronic Health Evaluation (APACHE) series — (APACHE IV validated in 2006.)

c) Describe the commonly used score in your intensive care unit and explain how you would use it. 2 marks

- APACHE II is commonly used in the UK still; it has only 17 variables.
- Provides a score of 0 to 71.
- Worst values over 24 hours are included.
- A score of 25 indicates a predicted mortality of 50%.
- A score of 35 or more indicates a predicted mortality of 80%.
- It is only an admission score and does not take into account any resuscitative or therapeutic efforts done before intensive care admission.

d) Why are early warning scores useful in acute illness and sepsis? 2 marks

- Timely recognition.
- Intervention and escalation of care.
- Improves patient outcomes and safety.

e) Give some examples of early intervention that could be offered if the early warning scores indicate the need. 2 marks

- Early antibiotics and infection source control in sepsis.
- Escalate care to the high dependency unit or intensive care unit.

f) List the advantages and limits of early warning scores. 2 marks

Advantages:

- A single physiologic parameter or several variables are combined to give an aggregate weighted score.
- Reflect acute illness severity.
- Common mode of communication among a range of health care professionals.
- Aim to escalate care in those at high risk.

Limits:

- User error.
- Inaccurate recording.
- Patients with chronic illness might already have abnormal results.
- Do not replace clinical judgement.

g) List the features used in the National Early Warning Score (NEWS). 3 mark

- A national standardised approach from the Royal College of Physicians (2012).
- Six physiogical variables — respiratory rate, SpO_2, temperature, systolic BP, heart rate, level of consciousness along with supplemental oxygen use.
- Urine output is excluded as this is not measured at the first assessment and not routinely measured.
- Superior to early warning scores.
- Refined in 2017 (NEWS2).

h) What are the ICNARC reports? 2 mark

- Intensive Care National Audit and Research Centre (ICNARC) — hospitals in England, Wales and Northern Ireland participate in the Case Mix Programme (CMP) and submit scoring system data over a time period; this helps to measure performance and compare with other intensive care units.
- Assist in decision-making, resource allocation and quality improvement.
- In Scotland, a similar process is led by the Scottish Intensive Care Society Quality Improvement Group (SICSQIG).
- The ICNARC score incorporates physiological, haematological, biochemical variables with age, severe chronic disease and circumstances related to intensive care admission.

i) What are the limitations of the ICNARC reports? 4 mark

- Limits related to scores to derive SMR (Standardised Mortality Ratio).
- Limits of unit comparison beyond scoring systems.
- Calibration of illness severity score weakens over time.
- APACHE II is not validated for children, or less than an 8-hour stay in the intensive care unit or readmissions.

- Excludes certain populations, e.g. burns, CABG, liver transplants.
- Do not correlate well with circumstances of admission.
- Overestimates the mortality risk for patients with DKA or major surgery with postoperative pain, or those under the effects of GA.
- Regional variations exist in the HDU and ICU.
- Not for highly specialised services, e.g. cardiac, ECMO, transplants.
- There is a selection bias as they do not include patients who are refused admission to the ICU.

References

1. Desai N, Gross J. Scoring systems in the critically ill: uses, cautions, and future directions. *Br J Anaesth Education* 2019; 19(7): 212-8.

Q15 — Long-term venous access

a) What are the main indications for long-term venous access? 3 mark

- Dialysis.
- Parenteral nutrition.
- Cancer therapy.
- Long-term antibiotic therapy.

b) What are the common types of long-term venous catheters? 4 mark

- Peripherally inserted central catheters (PICC).
- Midline catheters.
- Tunnelled cuffed catheters, e.g. Hickman.
- Port catheters.
- Dialysis catheters, e.g. Permcath™.

c) What are the main considerations for choosing the insertion site for long-term venous access? 4 mark

- Coagulopathy.
- Poor limb or vein condition.
- Musculoskeletal abnormalities.
- Comfortable site for long-term catheter.
- Cosmetic condition.
- Ease of maintenance of cleanliness.

d) What is the ideal site for catheter tip position? 4 mark

- Long axis of the superior vena cava.
- Upper right atrium outside the pericardial reflection.

e) What are the complications of long-term venous catheters? 5 marks

- Catheter occlusion.
- Extravasation.
- Catheter tip malposition.
- Phlebitis.
- Thrombosis.
- Catheter-related infection.
- Central vein stenosis.
- Catheter fracture.

References

1. Hudman L, Bodenham A. Practical aspects of long-term venous access. *Br J Anaesth CEACCP* 2013; 13(1): 6-11.
2. Moir M, Bodenham A. A narrative review of long-term central venous access devices for the intensivist. *Journal of the Intensive Care Society* 2018; 19(3): 236-46.

Q16 — ICU-acquired weakness

a) What are the main types of intensive care unit (ICU)-acquired weakness? 3 mar

- Critical illness polyneuropathy.
- Critical illness myopathy.
- Critical illness neuromyopathy.

b) What are the risk factors for ICU-acquired weakness? 4 mar

- Severe sepsis.
- Multi-organ failure.
- Prolonged mechanical ventilation.
- Long duration of SIRS.
- Hyperglycaemia.
- Female sex and old age.
- Malnutrition.
- Large cumulative dose of steroids.
- Prolonged neuromuscular blockade.
- Aminoglycosides.
- Renal replacement therapy.

c) What are the main postulated mechanisms in the development of ICU-acquired weakness? 4 mar

- Reduced oxygen delivery to the nerve axons.
- Mitochondrial dysfunction.
- Reduced nutrient delivery to the nerve axons.
- Altered membrane (sodium) channel function.
- Altered sarcoplasmic reticulum function in the release and uptake of calcium.
- Axonal damage from neurotoxins.
- Oxidative stress and damage secondary to hyperglycaemia.

- Muscle atrophy.
- Muscle denervation.

d) What are the main clinical features essential for diagnosing ICU-acquired weakness? 5 marks

- Weakness developing after an onset of critical illness.
- Generalised, symmetrical, flaccid weakness sparing cranial nerves.
- Cause of weakness not related to the underlying critical illness.
- Muscle power score fitting the criteria set by the Medical Research Council (MRC).
- Dependence on mechanical ventilation.

e) What are the main complications associated with ICU-acquired weakness? 2 marks

- Prolonged mechanical ventilation.
- The possibility of dangerous hyperkalaemia with depolarising neuromuscular blockers.
- Prolonged hospital length of stay.
- Increased morbidity and mortality.

f) What is the mainstay of treatment of ICU-acquired weakness? 2 marks

- Prevention.
- Rehabilitation.
- Physiotherapy.
- Occupational therapy.
- Psychological support.

References

1. Appleton R, Kinsella J. Intensive care unit-acquired weakness. *Br J Anaesth CEACCP* 2012; 12(2): 62-6.

Chapter 17

Perioperative medicine

ANSWERS

Q1 — Thyroidectomy

A patient presents for a total thyroidectomy.

a) Name any five specific investigations that are indicated in the preoperative assessment and explain why they are indicated. 5 marks

- Full blood count — to rule out the adverse effects of antithyroid medications such as thrombocytopenia; to measure baseline haemoglobin as total thyroidectomies can have significant blood loss.
- Thyroid function tests — the patient should be euthyroid prior to elective surgery to avoid the risk of a perioperative thyroid storm or myxoedema coma.
- Electrolytes and corrected calcium levels — to obtain baseline levels and rule out any calcium abnormalities.
- Chest X-ray:
  - to assess the size of the goitre;
  - to identify tracheal deviation/compression;
  - lateral thoracic inlet views to rule out retrosternal extension.
- CT scan of the airway — to delineate the extent of tracheal narrowing/invasion.
- Nasendoscopy — to record any pre-existing vocal cord dysfunction and/or laryngeal displacement.

b) What factors in a euthyroid patient must the anaesthetist consider during the induction and maintenance phases of a total thyroidectomy? 7 marks

Considerations during anaesthetic induction:

- Adequate preoxygenation and check the ability to ventilate prior to muscle relaxation.
- Consider spraying the vocal cords with lidocaine prior to intubation to reduce coughing on emergence.
- Avoid overinflating the tube cuff to minimise vocal cord/tracheal damage.
- If there are any concerns regarding the airway in the preoperative assessment, consider the following options:
  - inhalational induction with sevoflurane;
  - awake fibreoptic intubation;
  - tracheostomy under local anaesthetic performed by a surgeon;
  - ventilation through a rigid bronchoscope.

Considerations during the maintenance phase:

- Intravenous/inhalational maintenance with the use of a remifentanil infusion reduces the need for muscle relaxation and allows intraoperative electrophysiological monitoring of the recurrent laryngeal nerve, if required in complicated cases. It also provides a bloodless surgical field.
- Positioning with the head extended and sandbag under the shoulders for optimal surgical access.
- Eyes should be adequately padded especially in patients with exophthalmos.
- Avoid neck ties and maintain a head-up tilt to aid venous drainage.
- Maintain good access to an intravenous drip in the hands via long extensions.

- Analgesia with local infiltration by the surgeon and simple analgesia plus weak opioids.
- Multimodal antiemetics.

c) During extubation, what factors must be considered post-total thyroidectomy? 4 marks

- Assess haemostasis before wound closure by performing a Valsalva manoeuvre in a head-down position.
- If there are any concerns regarding the integrity of the recurrent laryngeal nerve, visualise the vocal cords with a laryngoscope or fibreoptic scope.
- Fully reverse neuromuscular blockade.
- Deflate the endotracheal tube cuff and ensure there is a leak around the tube prior to extubation, especially in large/longstanding goitres.
- Extubate the patient when awake and sitting upright.

d) List any four important postoperative complications following this surgery and how you would manage them. 4 marks

- Haemorrhage — may require the removal of surgical clips and re-exploration in the operating theatre.
- Laryngeal oedema — may occur as a result of traumatic intubation or with complex surgery. This is managed with corticosteroid therapy and humidified oxygen.
- Tracheomalacia — may occur in patients with large goitres/tumours; it requires immediate reintubation.
- Recurrent laryngeal nerve palsy — may occur due to ischaemia, traction, entrapment or transection of the nerve during surgery and may be unilateral or bilateral.
- Hypocalcaemia — temporary hypocalcaemia occurs in up to 20% of patients but permanent hypocalcaemia is rare. Calcium replacement (oral/intravenous) should be instituted immediately.

- Thyroid storm — less commonly seen as all patients are rendered euthyroid prior to elective surgery. Management is supportive with active cooling, hydration, beta-blockers and antithyroid drugs. Dantrolene has also been used successfully.

References

1. Malhotra S, Sodhi V. Anaesthesia for thyroid and parathyroid surgery. *Br J Anaesth CEACCP* 2007; 7(2): 55-8.
2. Adams L, Davies S. Anaesthesia for thyroid surgery. Anaesthesia tutorial of the week 162. https://www.wfsahq.org/components/com_virtual_library/media/4c4439eeda55fcfe86ddc98ca3980f30-bccc9b5455cac1cc0084a01c54dec630-162-Anaesthesia-for-thyroid-surgery.pdf. Accessed on 1st July 2019.

Q2 — Diabetes and anaesthesia

You are assessing a 63-year-old female for an elective laparotomy in the pre-anaesthetic assessment clinic. She has type I diabetes which is under control.

a) In a patient with diabetes mellitus, what clinical features may indicate autonomic involvement? 4 marks

- Cardiac autonomic neuropathy:
  - resting tachycardia and reduced heart rate variation;
  - orthostatic hypotension;
  - delayed recognition of ischaemic chest pain.
- Gastrointestinal autonomic neuropathy:
  - oesophageal dysfunction leading to heartburn and dysphagia;
  - delayed gastric emptying leading to early satiety, anorexia, nausea and vomiting;
  - small bowel dysfunction leading to alternating diarrhoea and constipation;
  - anal and rectal neuropathy;
  - gallbladder atony and enlargement.
- Genitourinary autonomic neuropathy:
  - neurogenic bladder;
  - sexual dysfunction.
- Hypoglycaemia unawareness.
- Anaemia due to reduced sympathetic stimulation of erythropoietin production.

b) What are the other microvascular and macrovascular complications of diabetes mellitus? 6 marks

Microvascular complications (due to tissue exposure to chronic hyperglycaemia):

- Nephropathy — commonest cause of renal failure in the developed world.
- Retinopathy — increased risk of retinal detachment, vitreous haemorrhage and macular oedema.
- Neuropathy — most common is a mixed sensory and motor polyneuropathy.
- Autonomic neuropathy.
- Focal neuropathies — carpal tunnel syndrome, third cranial nerve palsies, diabetic amyotrophy.

Macrovascular complications:

- Hypertension.
- Coronary artery disease.
- Cerebrovascular disease.
- Peripheral arterial disease.

c) List any five classes of oral hypoglycaemic agents that are available with an example. Describe the mechanism of action for each. 10 marks

Classes of oral hypoglycaemic agents:

- Sulphonylureas, e.g. tolbutamide, glibenclamide, gliclazide.
- Biguanides, e.g. metformin.
- Thiazolidinediones, e.g. pioglitazone.
- DPP-4 inhibitors, e.g. sitagliptin.
- Incretin agonists, e.g. exenatide.

- Meglitinides, e.g. repaglinide.
- Alpha-glucosidase inhibitors, e.g. acarbose.

Mechanisms of action:

- Sulphonylureas — stimulate insulin release from the pancreas and decrease insulin resistance in peripheral tissues (muscle and fat).
- Biguanides — decrease hepatic glucose output and increase insulin sensitivity at hepatic and peripheral tissues.
- Thiazolidinediones — improve peripheral uptake and utilisation of glucose in muscle and fat and also decrease liver glucose production.
- DPP-4 inhibitors — stimulate insulin secretion, inhibit glucagon secretion and preserve beta-cell mass in the pancreas.
- Incretin agonists — bind to glucagon-like peptide-1 (GLP-1) receptors, stimulate glucose-dependent insulin secretion, suppress glucagon secretion, slow gastric emptying and reduce food intake.
- Meglitinides — stimulate the release of insulin from the pancreatic beta cells.
- Alpha-glucosidase inhibitors — inhibit alpha-glucosidase, which converts complex carbohydrates into monosaccharides, thus, slowing and limiting the absorption of glucose.

References

1. Nicholson G, Hall GM. Diabetes and adult surgical inpatients. *Br J Anaesth CEACCP* 2011; 11(6): 234-8.

Q3 — Enhanced recovery programme

A 74-year-old patient is scheduled for a primary total hip replacement.

a) What are the advantages of an enhanced recovery programme (ERP) for this type of surgery? 5 marks

- Early mobilisation (operative day if possible).
- Reduced postoperative complications, especially cardiopulmonary.
- Earlier discharge.
- Theatre efficiency.
- Standardised care.
- Increased patient satisfaction.

b) What preoperative measures can be included in the ERP for this patient? 5 marks

- Patient education and engagement.
- Optimisation of comorbidities.
- Admission on the morning of surgery.
- Minimising fasting times and maintaining nutrition.
- Premedication to reduce the stress response, opioid requirements and improve analgesia. A combination of NSAIDs, gabapentin, paracetamol, clonidine and dexamethasone can be used.

c) List the intraoperative measures that can be included as part of the ERP in this case. 7 marks

- Judicious fluid management.
- Intraoperative use of tranexamic acid.
- Prevention of PONV, e.g. avoidance of nitrous oxide, use of TIVA, multimodal antiemetics.
- Regional anaesthesia — central neuraxial blocks without long-acting opioids.

- Local anaesthetic infiltration by surgeons with or without a nerve block.
- If using a general anaesthetic technique, the use of short-acting agents to quicken recovery times.
- Maintenance of normothermia.
- Surgical technique — minimise operative time, avoidance of drains.
- Avoidance of urinary catheters.

d) What postoperative measures can be included as part of the ERP for this patient? 3 marks

- Multimodal analgesia/oral opioids (avoid PCA).
- Encourage early oral intake (energy drinks).
- Planned early mobilisation and physiotherapy.

References

1. Place K, Scott NB. Enhanced recovery for lower limb arthroplasty. *Br J Anaesth CEACCP* 2014; 14(3): 95-9.

Q4 — Anaemia and anaesthesia

A 76-year-old patient who is scheduled for an elective primary total knee replacement is found to be anaemic, with a haemoglobin level of 90g/L.

a) List the perioperative consequences associated with preoperative anaemia. 5 marks

- Increased risk of 30-day postoperative mortality.
- Increased risk of cardiac events.
- Increased risk of major non-cardiac complications (respiratory, urinary, wound, septic and thromboembolic).
- Poor functional recovery/quality of life postoperatively.
- Increased length of hospital stay.
- Receipt of autologous red blood cells increases mortality and morbidity.

b) Name some physiological adaptations that can occur to offset the effects of anaemia. 5 marks

- Increased oxygen extraction by tissues such as the kidney, skeletal muscle and skin leading to an increased total oxygen extraction and reduced mixed venous oxygen saturation.
- Redistribution of cardiac output to organs with a high demand, i.e. brain and heart.
- Reduced blood viscosity leading to a decreased systemic vascular resistance and increased cardiac output.
- Rightward shift of the oxygen dissociation curve (due to a decrease in 2,3-DPG and hydrogen ions) causes a reduced affinity of haemoglobin for oxygen and favours its release at higher partial pressures.
- Reduced oxygen tension triggers the transcription of hypoxia-response genes, such as erythropoietin and vascular endothelium growth factor.

c) List any five perioperative events that may worsen the effects of anaemia. 5 marks

Increased oxygen demand:

- Pain.
- Fever.
- Shivering.
- Stress response.

Reduced oxygen supply:

- Atelectasis, pneumonia, thromboembolic events.
- Hypovolaemia.
- Cardiac depression by anaesthetic agents.
- Haemorrhage.
- Hypothermia leading to a left shift of the oxygen dissociation curve.

d) List further blood tests that may help to classify this anaemia. 5 marks

- Reticulocyte count.
- Mean corpuscular volume.
- Ferritin level.
- Transferrin saturation.
- Urea and electrolytes.
- Liver function tests.
- Inflammatory markers.
- Vitamin B12 levels.
- Folate levels.
- LDH.
- Serum iron.
- Free plasma haemoglobin.
- Haptoglobin.

References

1. Hans GA, Jones N. Preoperative anaemia. *Br J Anaesth CEACCP* 2013; 13(3): 71-4.

Q5 — CPET testing

a) List the main measures of fitness obtained by CPET testing and explain what it is. 4 marks

The main measures of fitness obtained by CPET testing are:

- Peak oxygen uptake (VO_2 peak):
  - measure of maximal exercise capacity for the patient;
  - defined as the highest oxygen uptake at end-exercise on a rapid incremental test;
  - measured in ml/min or ml/kg/min.
- Anaerobic threshold (AT):
  - oxygen consumption for a patient at which anaerobic metabolism starts supplementing the aerobic metabolism;
  - measured in ml/min or ml/kg/min.
- Ventilatory equivalents ($VE/VECO_2$):
  - ratio of minute ventilation to CO_2 output;
  - measure of ventilatory efficiency.

b) List any four abnormalities on CPET testing that indicate cardiorespiratory disease with the values. 4 marks

- Anaerobic threshold </= 11ml/kg/min.
- Peak oxygen uptake </=15ml/kg/min.
- VO_2 max or peak <84% predicted.
- Anaerobic threshold <40% VO_2 max predicted.
- Vitals range — heart rate, BP, respiratory rate.
- Ventilatory reserve (VR) = MVV-VEmax <11L/min.
- VE/VCO_2 >34.
- PaO_2 <80mmHg.
- $P(A\text{-}a)O_2$ >35mmHg.

c) What are the indications for CPET testing? 3 marks

- To estimate perioperative mortality and morbidity and contribute to the preoperative risk assessment.
- To contribute towards multidisciplinary shared decision-making and consent.
- To predict the most appropriate level of care postoperatively.

d) List other tests to assess the patient's functional capacity. 3 marks

- Incremental shuttle walk test.
- 6-minute walk test.
- Stair climb test.

e) What scoring systems can help to predict perioperative risk before major non-cardiac surgery? 6 marks

- P-POSSUM.
- Surgical Outcome Risk Tool (SORT).
- American College of Surgeons National Surgical Quality Improvement Program (ACS NSQIP) risk calculator score.
- Surgical Risk Scale (SRS).
- Acute Physiology and Chronic Health Evaluation (APACHE 2) score.
- American Society of Anesthesiologists Physical Status (ASA-PS) score.

References

1. Agnew N. Preoperative cardiopulmonary exercise testing. *Br J Anaesth CEACCP* 2010; 10(2): 33-7.
2. Schonborn JL, Anderson H. Perioperative medicine: a changing model of care. *Br J Anaesth Education* 2019; 19(1): 27-33.

3. Levett DZH, Jack S, Swart M, *et al*. Perioperative cardiopulmonary testing (CPET): consensus clinical guidelines on indications, organization, conduct, and physiological interpretation. *Br J Anaesth* 2017; 120(3): 484-500.

Q6 — Prehabilitation

a) What is prehabilitation in perioperative medicine? 1 mark

Prehabilitation is the practice of enhancing a patient's functional capacity before surgery, with the aim of improving postoperative outcomes.

b) What are the outcome benefits of a prehabilitation programme? 3 mark

- Improvement in length of hospital stay.
- Reduced postoperative pain.
- Improvement in postoperative outcomes.

c) Which specific issues are addressed as part of medical optimisation in a prehabilitation programme? 6 mark

- Preoperative smoking cessation.
- Reduced alcohol intake.
- Weight optimisation.
- Management of anaemia.
- Control of blood glucose.
- Optimisation of pharmacological therapy.

d) How would a prehabilitation exercise program improve a patient's cardiorespiratory reserve? 4 mark

The response to exercise training causes:

- Increased cardiac output, arteriovenous oxygen difference and VO_2 max.
- Skeletal muscle adaptations — increased mitochondrial content and oxygen uptake capacity.

- Overall functional reserve increases to meet the increased metabolic demands of surgery and the postoperative period.

e) What are the benefits of carbohydrate preloading and nutritional optimisation? 4 marks

The benefits of carbohydrate preloading:

- Reduces insulin resistance.
- Promotes an anabolic state.
- Minimises the loss of protein, lean body mass and muscle function.

Nutritional optimisation with immunonutrition, ingestion of amino acids, omega 3 fatty acids and nucleotides:

- Counteracts hyperinflammation and immune impairment.
- Promotes wound healing.
- Reduces infection rates.
- Shortens hospital length of stay.

f) What psychologically supportive interventions may be used in prehabilitation? 2 marks

- Providing sensory information (what the perioperative experience will feel like).
- Cognitive intervention such as the development of a positive attitude.
- Behavioural instruction.
- Relaxation techniques such as hypnosis and muscle relaxation techniques.
- Providing procedural information.
- Emotion-focused intervention.

References

1. Banugo P, Amoako D. Prehabilitation. *Br J Anaesth Education* 2017; 17(2): 401-5.

Q7 — Scoring systems in anaesthesia

a) Describe the risk assessment tools commonly used in anaesthesia. 2 marks

- ASA Physical Status (ASA-PS) score.
- Cardiac Risk Index.
- Respiratory risk scores.
- POSSUM, P-POSSUM.
- NELA calculator.
- EuroSCORE.

b) Name and describe a risk score for cardiac complications. 2 marks

- Lee's Revised Cardiac Risk Index (RCRI).
- This is the most commonly used risk score for cardiac complications after major non-cardiac surgeries.
- There are six independent predictors — high-risk surgery, ischaemic heart disease, CCF, CVA, insulin therapy, creatinine >176μmol/L.
- There are four classes— class 1 has a 0.1% risk but class 4 has an 11% risk.

c) Name and detail a risk score for postoperative pulmonary complications. 2 marks

- Assess Respiratory risk In Surgical patients in CATalonia (ARIS-CAT) score.
- This is a seven-variable risk model — age, SpO_2, respiratory infection in the last month, preop Hb <100g/L, surgical incision site, duration of surgery, emergency procedure.

d) What are the components of the POSSUM and P-POSSUM risk prediction models? 6 mark

- POSSUM — Physiological and Operative Severity Score for the enUmeration of Mortality and morbidity.
- There are 12 physiological variables and six surgical variables.
- Calculates the 30-day mortality after surgery.
- The physiological variables are — age, cardiac signs, respiratory rate, systolic BP, heart rate, GCS, Hb, WBC, urea, sodium, potassium, ECG.
- Operative variables are — severity, multiple procedures, blood loss, peritoneal soiling, malignancy, urgency of surgery.
- P-POSSUM — Portsmouth POSSUM.
- P-POSSUM uses alternative risk equations, but the same variables.
- Comprehensive and well validated.

e) What is the NELA calculator and what does it estimate? 2 mark

- It estimates 30-day mortality after emergency bowel surgery.
- The P-POSSUM model is used to predict mortality, but it is overestimated if the risk is >15%.
- The NELA calculator is accurate and specific for emergency laparotomies.
- It is time consuming, requires intraoperative findings, and does not give morbidity.

f) The NCEPOD enquiry in 2011 produced the SORT tool; list any four variables that are used in this tool. 2 mark

- SORT tool — Surgical Outcome Risk Tool.
- There are six preoperative variables — ASA-PS, urgency, specialty, severity, cancer, age.
- It predicts 30-day mortality in non-cardiac, non-neurological inpatient surgery.

g) Outline the difference between risk scores and risk prediction models. 4 marks

- Risk assessment tools can be divided into risk scores and risk prediction models; both are developed with multivariable analysis of risk factors leading to a specific outcome.
- Risk scores assign a weighting to factors identified as independent predictors of an outcome; this allows comparison with other patients on a scale. They are simple to use.
- Risk prediction models estimate the individual probability of risk by entering the patient's data into the model. They are more accurate in predicting, but are more complex for routine use.

References

1. Stones J, Yates D. Clinical risk assessment tools in anaesthesia. *Br J Anaesth Education* 2019; 19(2): 47-53.

Chapter 18

Regional, orthopaedic and trauma anaesthesia

ANSWERS

Q1 — Nerve block for shoulder surgery

a) List the specific nerves that need to be blocked to achieve effective analgesia for shoulder surgery. 6 marks

The shoulder area is supplied by both the cervical and brachial plexus as follows:

Cervical plexus:

- Transverse cervical nerve.
- Supraclavicular nerve.

Brachial plexus:

- Upper lateral cutaneous branch of the axillary nerve.
- Medial cutaneous nerve of the arm.
- Intercostobrachial nerve.
- Suprascapular nerve.

b) Name any six possible complications of an interscalene block. 6 marks

- Subarachnoid/epidural injection.
- Stellate ganglion block.
- Pneumothorax.
- Phrenic nerve palsy — ipsilateral hemidiaphragmatic paralysis.
- Horner's syndrome.
- Local anaesthetic toxicity.
- Accidental intravenous injection.

c) What positioning is needed for shoulder surgery? 1 mark

The deck chair (modified sitting position) is most commonly used for shoulder surgeries.

d) List any three complications of positioning for shoulder surgery. 3 marks

- Hypotension due to venous pooling in the extremities.
- Intraoperative cerebral ischaemia.
- Activation of the Bezold-Jarisch reflex leading to profound bradycardia, hypotension and even cardiac arrest.
- Neurological injuries.

e) What postoperative advice would you give to a patient who has received an interscalene block? 4 marks

- After an interscalene block, your arm may remain weak for up to 24 hours.
- As the numbness wears off, it is normal to feel pins and needles in the hand.
- Take regular analgesics postoperatively to avoid sudden intense pain once the block wears off.

- Protect and support your arm, preferably in a sling.
- Avoid handling machinery, driving, and contact with very hot or cold objects.
- If the numbness lasts for more than 24 hours or you get breathless, ring the hospital number provided.

References

1. Beecroft CL, Coventry DM. Anaesthesia for shoulder surgery. *Br J Anaesth CEACCP* 2008; 8(6): 193-8.
2. Hewson DW, Oldman M, Bedforth NM. Regional anaesthesia for shoulder surgery. *Br J Anaesth Education* 2019; 19(4): 98-104.

Q2 — Regional block in hip fractures

An 80-year-old woman is admitted to hospital having sustained a proximal femoral (neck of femur) fracture in a fall.

a) How would you optimise this patient's pain preoperatively? 5 mark

- Assessment of pain by recording pain scores should be done on admission to the accident and emergency department, after 30 minutes and then regularly after starting regular analgesia.
- Immobilisation of the injured leg.
- Simple analgesia with paracetamol (avoid NSAIDs).
- Multimodal analgesia with sparing use of opioids.
- Regional nerve blocks.

b) What is the nerve supply of the skin overlying the hip joint? 5 mark

- Cluneal nerves — superior, medial and inferior.
- Anterior cutaneous branch of the femoral nerve.
- Cutaneous branch of the obturator nerve.
- Lateral cutaneous nerve of the thigh.
- Lateral cutaneous branch of the iliohypogastric nerve.

c) What regional nerve blocks can be used to provide preoperative analgesia? 2 mark

- Femoral nerve block.
- Fascia iliaca block.
- Lateral cutaneous nerve of the thigh block.
- Psoas block.

d) What nerves are blocked by the fascia iliaca block? 2 marks

- Lateral femoral cutaneous nerve.
- Femoral nerve.
- Obturator nerve.

e) List the scoring systems that can be used to predict 30-day mortality in this patient. 2 marks

- Nottingham Hip Fracture Score.
- Estimation of Physiological Ability and Surgical Stress (E-PASS).
- O-POSSUM (Physiological and Operative Severity Score for the enUmeration of Mortality and morbidity modified for orthopaedic usage).

f) List the AAGBI recommendations regarding unacceptable reasons for delaying surgery. 4 marks

- Lack of facilities or operating theatre space.
- Awaiting echocardiography.
- Unavailable surgical expertise.
- Minor electrolyte abnormalities.

References

1. Maxwell L, White S. Anaesthetic management of patients with hip fractures: an update. *Br J Anaesth CEACCP* 2013; 13(5): 179-83.

Q3 — Ultrasound

a) Outline the basic physical principles involved in the formation of an ultrasound image. 1 mark

The formation of an ultrasound image is based upon sound waves that are transmitted from, and received by, an US transducer. It utilises frequencies of 2-15MHz (human hearing operates at 1-20kHz).

b) What is piezoelectrical activity and how is it utilised in ultrasound? 2 mark

Ultrasound transducers have piezoelectric properties:

- When current is applied across the crystal, it expands and contracts as the polarity of the voltage changes. This produces a series of pressure waves (sound waves).
- In reverse, when the sound wave returns, it squeezes and stretches the crystal and generates a voltage change across its surface. This is amplified and forms the receiving signal.

c) What governs the reflection of sound waves and the formation of an ultrasound image? 2 mark

- The reflectivity of sound waves depends on the difference in the acoustic impedance of the two media at an interface.
- The higher the difference in acoustic impedance, the greater the reflection, thus obscuring the deeper tissues, e.g. a tissue-air interface has a reflection coefficient of 0.999 and 99% of the sound waves are reflected.

d) List the patient factors that influence ultrasound image quality. 4 marks

- Increased Body Mass Index.
- Tissue oedema.
- Muscle atrophy.
- Anatomical abnormalities.

e) What acoustic artefacts may influence the ultrasound image quality? 4 marks

- Postcystic enhancement — fluid-filled structures like a cyst provide increased brightness behind them.
- Acoustic shadowing — caused by highly reflective surfaces such as bone.
- Anisotropy — image quality is affected by the angle at which the ultrasound beam hits the target.
- Air — air does not allow the passage of ultrasound beams.

f) Which two needling techniques are commonly used in ultrasound-guided nerve blocks? 2 marks

- In-plane needling technique or long-axis technique.
- Out-of-plane needling technique or short-axis technique.

g) List the advantages and disadvantages of one of these techniques. 5 marks

In-plane needling technique:

- Advantages:
  - able to visualise the entire length of the needle;
  - able to visualise the proximity of the nerve to the needle.

- Disadvantages:
  - difficulty in keeping the needle in view;
  - the needle entry point may be unusual;
  - longer distance from the skin entry point to the nerve.

References

1. Carty S, Nicholls B. Ultrasound-guided regional anaesthesia. *Br J Anaesth CEACCP* 2007; 7(1): 20-4.

Q4 — Spinal cord transection injury

A 19-year-old patient has suffered a complete transection of the spinal cord at the first thoracic vertebral level due to a fall but has no other injuries.

a) What is the pathophysiology of neurological injury subsequent to the fall in this patient? 3 marks

Primary injury:

- From direct cord compression.
- Haemorrhage.
- Traction forces.

Secondary injury:

- Haemorrhage in the central grey matter damages the axons and neuronal cell membrane.
- This leads to spinal cord oedema and subsequent spinal cord ischaemia.
- Loss of autoregulation contributes to neurogenic shock.
- A persistent drop in the systemic arterial pressure may lead to further cord hypoperfusion causing a spread in the damaged zone (penumbra).
- Cord ischaemia extends bidirectionally.
- Secondary spinal cord injury ensues further.

b) What is the cause of neurogenic shock in this patient and how does it present? 1 mark

Neurogenic shock — interruption of autonomic pathways leading to hypotension and bradycardia.

c) How would spinal shock present in this patient and what are the phases? 2 mar

Spinal shock:

- Loss of reflexes below the level of the spinal cord injury.
- Results in the clinical signs of flaccid areflexia.
- Usually combined with hypotension of neurogenic shock.

Stages of spinal shock:

- Areflexia (days 0-1).
- Initial reflex return (days 1-3).
- Early hyperreflexia (days 4-28).
- Late hyperreflexia (1-12 months).

d) What disturbances may occur subsequently in the cardiovascular system? 4 mar

- An initial massive release of catecholamines leads to dramatic hypertension and tachycardia.
- A loss of sympathetic tone leads to vasodilatation and hypotension.
- Bradycardia from unopposed vagal tone also contributes to hypotension as does negative inotropism.
- Pulmonary capillary integrity is lost which predisposes this patient to pulmonary oedema.

e) What effects may be seen in the respiratory system? 4 mar

- Loss of inspiratory intercostal muscle and abdominal muscle contribution to the work of breathing.
- Vital capacity reduced to 30-80% of normal.
- Normal to weak cough.
- Short-term ventilation may be needed.

- Long-term ventilation may be needed if the patient has other comorbidities.

f) When and why may suxamethonium be contraindicated in this patient? 2 marks

- Suxamethonium should be avoided from 72 hours post-injury and for up to 6 months after the injury.
- Acute denervation causes the development of extrajunctional acetylcholine receptors. Due to this, the use of suxamethonium in this patient can lead to life-threatening hyperkalaemia.

g) Give the advantages of a regional anaesthetic technique for a patient having elective lower limb surgery 2 years after a high thoracic spine transection. 4 marks

This patient may safely have a spinal anaesthetic for elective lower limb surgery 2 years post-spinal cord injury.

Advantages:

- Abolishes autonomic dysreflexia.
- Avoids the development of spasms perioperatively.
- Reduces the incidence of thromboembolism.
- Avoids the risks from airway manipulation for general anaesthesia.
- Avoids the need for ventilation in this patient who may already have respiratory compromise due to the spinal cord injury.

References

1. Bonner S, Smith C. Initial management of acute spinal cord injury. *Br J Anaesth CEACCP* 2013; 13(6): 224-31.
2. Petsas A, Drake J. Perioperative management for patients with a chronic spinal cord injury. *Br J Anaesth Education* 2015; 15(3): 123-30.

Q5 — Wrong-side block and never events

a) List the implications for the patient of an inadvertent wrong-sided peripheral nerve block. 5 marks

- Nerve injury from siting the wrong block.
- Local anaesthetic toxicity while siting the block.
- Delayed hospital discharge from reduced mobility.
- Implications for the patient's dexterity.
- May lead the team to continue with the wrong-site surgery.

b) Summarise the recommendations of the "Stop Before You Block" campaign. 5 marks

- Perform the WHO checklist sign in as usual.
- Extra vigilance under the following circumstances:
  - delay between sign in and doing the actual block;
  - when the patient has been moved/turned;
  - the presence of distractions in the anaesthetic room;
  - when performing lower limb blocks;
  - when less experienced personnel are performing the block.
- The anaesthetist and anaesthetic assistant should perform a "STOP" moment just before needle insertion. The surgical site marking and the site of the block should be confirmed.

c) List the factors that have been identified as contributing to the performance of a wrong-side block. 3 marks

- Distractions in the anaesthetic room.
- Time lag between the WHO sign in and the siting of the block.
- Covering up of the surgical marking with blankets to avoid the patient getting cold.

d) Define the term "never event". 2 mar

Never events are defined as "serious, largely preventable patient safety incidents that should not occur if relevant preventive measures have been put in place".

e) List any five drug-related never events. 5 mar

- Mis-selection of a strong potassium solution.
- Administration of medication by the wrong route.
- Overdose of insulin due to abbreviations or an incorrect device.
- Overdose of methotrexate for non-cancer treatment.
- Mis-selection of high-strength midazolam during conscious sedation.

References

1. Adyanthaya SS, Patil V. Never events: an anaesthetic perspective. *Br J Anaesth CEACCP* 2014; 14(5): 197-201.
2. Stop Before you Block Campaign. Safe Anaesthesia Liaison Group: NHS England; Nottingham University Hospitals NHS Trust; Regional Anaesthesia — United Kingdom. https://www.rcoa.ac.uk/sites/default/files/CSQ-PS-sbyb-supporting.pdf. Accessed on 25th June 2019.
3. The never events policy framework. Department of Health.
4. Never events list 2018. NHS improvement.

Q6 — Ankle block

A 32-year-old patient is scheduled for hallux valgus surgery.

a) What anaesthetic options are available for anaesthetising this patient? 3 marks

- General anaesthesia.
- Regional anaesthesia:
  - spinal anaesthesia;
  - popliteal sciatic block;
  - ankle block.
- A combination of the above techniques.

b) List the nerves supplying the ankle joint. 5 marks

- Posterior tibial nerve.
- Deep peroneal nerve.
- Superficial peroneal nerve.
- Saphenous nerve.
- Sural nerve.

c) Describe the origin and sensory innervation from the posterior tibial nerve. 3 marks

Posterior tibial nerve:

- Terminal branch of the tibial nerve.
- Mixed sensory and motor nerve.
- Enters the foot posterior to the medial malleolus.
- Commonly lies posterior to the posterior tibial vessels.
- Divides into medial and lateral plantar branches.
- Supplies the majority of the sole of the foot.

d) Describe the origin and sensory innervation from the deep peroneal nerve. 3 marks

Deep peroneal nerve:

- Branch of the common peroneal nerve.
- Enters the foot underneath the extensor retinaculum between the tendons of extensor digitorum longus and extensor hallucis longus.
- Lies lateral to the dorsalis pedis artery.
- Supplies the skin of the first web space.

e) Describe the origin and sensory innervation from the superficial peroneal nerve. 3 marks

Superficial peroneal nerve:

- Branch of the common peroneal nerve.
- Enters the superficial fascia in the dorsal aspect of the foot after piercing the deep fascia between extensor digitorum longus and peroneus brevis.
- Sensory to the majority of the dorsum of the foot.

f) List the disadvantages of using an ankle block for this patient. 3 marks

- Multiple injections may be uncomfortable especially if the patient is awake.
- An inability to use a proximal tourniquet for an extended duration.
- Time consuming.
- Risk of vascular injection.
- Failure/inadequate block.

References

1. Purushothaman L, Allan AGL, Bedforth N. Ultrasound-guided ankle block. *Br J Anaesth CEACCP* 2013; 13(5): 174-8.

Q7 — Pelvic fractures

You are called to resuscitate a 26-year-old male who had a major accident while driving a motorcycle. He is diagnosed with a pelvic fracture.

a) How would you classify pelvic fractures? 4 mark

The Young and Burgess classification (based on the direction of force causing the injury):

- AP compression — head-on collision; the pubic symphysis widens.
- Lateral compression — hit from one side; internal rotation of one side of the pelvis and anterior pubic rami fracture.
- Vertical shear — fall from height or axial loading of an extended limb on collision; complete disruption of the pelvic ring with superior displacement of the hemipelvis.
- A combined mechanism — a combination of the above forces.

Pelvic ring fractures can be stable or unstable:

- Stable — low-energy mechanism of injury, heals well.
- Unstable — secondary to a high-impact injury, associated with haemorrhage; two types:
  - with rotational instability only;
  - with rotational and vertical instability.

b) How would you initially manage and resuscitate this patient? 6 mark

- ATLS® approach — ABCDE approach.
- Mostly presents to major trauma centres.
- Team approach.
- Identify and manage life-threatening injuries.
- Pelvic binder application, and skeletal traction if there is also vertical instability.

- Usually multiple injuries have been sustained — care in assessing and managing.
- Do not stress the pelvis mechanically as it can destabilise clot formation.
- Avoid log rolling.
- Haemodynamic stability determines what radiological investigations could be undertaken.
- CT scan or contrast CT scan.
- If the patient is unresponsive to resuscitation, rapid intervention is needed with multi-specialty involvement and consultant-led decision-making.
- The immediate options are angiography and embolisation if available, or pelvic packing after an emergency laparotomy.
- Analgesia — IV morphine titrated; ketamine can be used as a second-line analgesic. Intranasal diamorphine can be used if there is no IV access.
- Bleeding should be controlled.

c) How would you apply a pelvic binder in this patient and how long would you leave it? 2 marks

- The early use of a pelvic binder improves the outcome.
- The aim is to approximate the fracture ends, to reduce bleeding, to reduce pain and to stabilise the pelvis temporarily.
- The binder can be placed over the greater trochanters, making sure there is exposure available if a laparotomy is needed.
- The disadvantages of using a pelvic binder are that it will not reduce vertical displacement and it can worsen the deformity in lateral compression fractures. It can also cause pressure sores, nerve damage, tissue necrosis, etc.
- Remove within 24 hours of application (NICE NG37, 2016).

d) What are the surgical options that are available in this patient? 2 mark

Surgical stabilisation/fixation in two stages:

- Initial stabilisation.
- Definitive fixation.

Stabilisation:

- External fixator.
- Skeletal traction.
- Pelvic packing.
- Radiological embolisation, etc.

Fixation:

- Approach to the anterior ring — common, pubic diastasis plate.
- Approach to the posterior ring — posterior ilium, sacrum.
- Approach to the acetabulum — anterior or posterior column.

e) What are the anaesthetic considerations in this patient with a traumatic pelvic fracture? 6 mark

Preoperative:

- Communication, MDT approach.
- Urological input.
- Prepare cell salvage, correct coagulopathy and cross-match for red cells.
- Electrolyte abnormalities corrected.
- Book a critical care bed.

Intraoperative:

- Two large-bore IV cannulae.
- Arterial line.
- Full AAGBI monitoring.
- Reinforced tracheal tube if a prone posture is used.
- Take care not to dislodge any chest drains, suprapubic catheters, extraventricular drains, etc.
- Prophylactic antibiotics.
- Tranexamic acid 1g loading dose and 1g infusion.
- Active mechanical compression devices for preventing VTE.

Postoperative:

- Multimodal analgesia.
- Local wound infiltration.
- Epidural analgesia (if continuous passive motion devices are used in acetabular surgeries).
- Intensive or high dependency care unit.

Thromboprophylaxis:

- Mechanical prophylaxis as soon as admitted.
- Chemical prophylaxis once haemodynamically stable, clotting corrected.
- If a high-risk patient, consider a IVC filter prophylactically.

References

1. Akuji MA, Chapman EE, Clements PAD. Anaesthesia for the management of traumatic pelvic fractures. *Br J Anaesth Education* 2018; 18(7): 204-10.
2. Fractures (complex): assessment and management. NICE guideline, NG37. London: National Institute for Health and Care Excellence, 2016, 2017. https://www.nice.org.uk/guidance/ng37. Accessed on 12th July 2019.

Q8 — Bone cement syndrome

A 78-year-old patient is undergoing an elective total hip replacement.

a) During the surgery, when can the patient present with bone cement implantation syndrome (BCIS)? 3 marks

- At the time of cementation.
- Insertion of prosthesis.
- Reduction of joint.
- Limb tourniquet deflation.

b) What clinical features would make you suspect a BCIS? 1 mark

- Transient/sustained desaturation.
- Hypotension.
- Cardiac arrhythmias.
- Cardiac arrest.

c) How would you grade the severity of BCIS? 3 marks

- Grade 1 — moderate hypoxia (SaO_2 <94%) or a reduction in systolic arterial pressure of >20%.
- Grade 2 — severe hypoxia (SaO_2 <88%) or a reduction in systolic arterial pressure of >40%) or unexpected unconsciousness.
- Grade 3 — cardiovascular collapse needing CPR.

d) What is the pathophysiology of BCIS? 4 marks

There are two probable theories:

- Mechanical effects — high intramedullary pressure causes embolisation of debris (marrow, fat, cement particles, air, bone particles, platelet aggregates, fibrin aggregates) to the right atrium/right ventricle/pulmonary artery. This leads to an increased pulmonary vascular resistance (PVR).

- Mediator effects — systemic embolisation of bone cement causes release of vasoactive/pro-inflammatory mediators which directly increase the PVR.

Increased PVR leads to a ventilation-perfusion mismatch, thus leading to hypoxia.

e) What are the risk factors for the development of BCIS? 5 marks

Patient-associated risk factors:

- ASA III or IV.
- Significant cardiovascular disease.
- Pre-existing pulmonary vascular hypertension.
- Osteoporosis.

Surgical risk factors:

- Aetiology of fracture — pathological fracture.
- Site of fracture — intertrochanteric fracture.
- Type of prosthesis — long-stem arthroplasty.

f) How can surgeons minimise the risk of development of BCIS? 4 marks

- Consider using a cementless hip prosthesis.
- Adequate lavage of the intramedullary canal of the shaft of the femur to ensure removal of debris.
- Ensure good haemostasis.
- Drilling a venting hole on the distal shaft of the femur to act as a pressure relieving opening during intramedullary reaming.
- The use of a bone-vacuum cementing technique.
- Retrograde insertion of cement by a cement gun.

References

1. Khanna G, Cernovsky J. Bone cement and the implications for anaesthesia. *Br J Anaesth CEACCP* 2012; 12(4): 213-6.

Q9 — Nerve injury after a regional block

You are part of the in-patient pain ward round. You are asked by ward staff to review a 38-year-old female who had a femoral nerve block followed by general anaesthesia for an external fixator of her lower leg 2 days ago. She complains of symptoms related to nerve injury in the particular dermatome since the nerve block.

a) What is the incidence of peripheral nerve injury after surgery? 1 mark

- 3 in 10,000.
- Peripheral nerve injury is nine times more related to surgical or patient factors rather than to a nerve block.
- Persistence of symptoms — 0-2.2% at 3 months, 0-0.8% at 6 months, 0-0.2% at 1 year.

b) Explain the anatomy of peripheral nerves in general. 3 marks

- Peripheral nerves — numerous fascicles are held together by connective tissue epineurium.
- Perineurium — multilayered epithelial sheath around each fascicle.
- Inside each fascicle, axons and capillary blood vessels are embedded in the endoneurium.
- Vasa nervorum — blood supply (extrinisic and intrinsic).

c) How would you classify the severity of nerve injury? 2 marks

Seddon classification — according to disruption of the axon:

- Neuropraxia — damage limited to the myelin sheath only; the best prognosis.
- Axonotmesis — intact endoneurium, but loss of axonal continuity.
- Neurotmesis — complete transection of the nerve, usually requiring surgical intervention; the worst prognosis.

d) What are the mechanisms of nerve injury? 2 mark

Four categories:

- Mechanical.
- Pressure.
- Chemical.
- Vascular.

Anaesthetic, surgical and patient factors:

- Anaesthetic — needle placement, pressure of injection, chemical and additives.
- Surgical — patient positioning, traction, stretch, compression, ischaemia, contusion, transection, post-surgical inflammatory neuropathy, double-crush theory (already susceptible patients).
- Patient — metabolic (diabetes), entrapment, toxic, hereditary, demyelination, ischaemic neuropathies, anticoagulant therapy, peripheral vascular disease, smoking, hypertension, vasculitis.

e) What factors would you consider to reduce nerve injury in your practice? 4 mark

- Nerve localisation techniques — triple monitoring — nerve stimulation, ultrasound and pressure monitoring.
- Paraesthesia is not reliable, but if elicited, the injection should be stopped.
- Peripheral nerve stimulation — a current intensity of 0.2-0.5mA with a pulse duration of 0.1ms is safe for placement of local anaesthetic — it is not reliable and nerve damage could already have occurred.
- Electrical impedance — extraneural vs. intraneural components.
- Ultrasound — visualisation of spread, reduced dose need, decreased intravascular puncture, reduced local anaesthetic systemic toxicity (LAST).

- Injection pressure monitoring — highly sensitive for an intrafascicular intraneural injection, but lacks specificity; <15psi indicates an extrafascicular injection.
- Equipment-related factors:
  - needle design — blunt short bevelled needles (45°) cause less trauma;
  - adjuvants — avoid neurotoxic additives; amides are safer. Ropivacaine has the lowest potential for neurotoxicity. Local mediated vasoconstriction occurs more often with levobupivacaine than lignocaine.
- Patient selection — avoid metabolic or neuropathic conditions.
- Awake better than asleep.

f) How would you evaluate the above patient and what diagnostic tests could be used? 2 marks

- Early recognition and prompt risk stratification to prioritise those needing urgent attention (imaging +/- neurological consultation).
- Early surgical and/or medical consultation to be sought.
- Patient evaluation — a thorough history and examination.
- Rule out other signs of infection (especially if a catheter is inserted).
- Diagnostic tests — neurophysiological studies to assess the function of nerves and muscles — EMG, NCS or both.

g) How would you manage this patient? Explain the RA-UK guidelines where appropriate in this management plan. 6 marks

Mild or resolving symptoms or sensory deficits:

- Reassure the patient and review in 4 weeks.
- If persistent refer to neurology; consider MRI and other imaging, NCS, EMG.
- Definitive diagnosis, treatment, surgery, informing the patient and team, follow-up.

Complete or progressive neurological deficit or the presence of motor deficit:

- Surgical cause to be assessed and intervention as appropriate (e.g. haematoma, cut, stretch injury — decompression, reconstruction, etc.).
- Further imaging and intervention (e.g. space-occupying lesion).
- Immediate neurological referral.
- NCS, EMG.
- Definitive diagnosis, treatment — drugs, physiotherapy, etc.
- Surgical intervention if required.
- Follow-up as appropriate.

References

1. O'Flaherty D, McCartney CJL, Ng SC. Nerve injury after peripheral nerve blockade — current understanding and guidelines. *Br J Anaesth Education* 2018, 18(12): 384-90.
2. RA-UK guidelines for supervision of patients during peripheral regional anaesthesia. Regional Anaesthesia — United Kingdom, 2015. https://www.ra-uk.org/images/Documents/RA-UK_guidelines_for_supervision_of_patients_during_peripheral_regional_anaesthesia.pdf. Accessed on 25th July 2019.

Q10 — Local anaesthetic toxicity

a) What are the clinical features of local anaesthetic systemic toxicity (LAST)? 4 marks

Neurological:

- Two stages — an initial excitatory phase followed by a depressive phase.
- Perioral tingling, tinnitus, slurred speech, lightheadedness, tremor, agitation.
- Toxicity can occur without these symptoms also.
- Generalised convulsions.
- Coma, respiratory depression.

Cardiovascular:

- Three phases.
- Initial hypertension, tachycardia.
- Intermediate — hypotension.
- Terminal phase — peripheral vasodilatation, fall in BP severe, arrhythmias, asystole.

b) What are the mechanisms of LAST? 2 marks

- Systemic absorption or accidental IV injection.
- Lipophilic local anaesthetic.
- Crosses the cell membrane and causes toxicity — various sites including inotropic, metabotropic and other targets.
- Affects balance between excitatory and inhibitory pathways.
- Conduction blocks on sodium, potassium and calcium channels.
- Disrupts signals at metabotropic receptors, reduced cyclic AMP concentration, reduced contractility.

c) What are the risk factors for LAST? 6 marks

Related to local anaesthetic:

- Type of local — bupivacaine is more toxic than levobupivacaine; levobupivacaine and ropivacaine have vasoconstrictor effects; the CC/CNS ratio is the ratio to produce cardiovascular collapse to that needed for seizures — bupivacaine has a ratio of 2 whereas lignocaine has a ratio of 7.
- Dose of local — the maximum dose of bupivacaine is 2mg/kg and for lignocaine this is 3mg/kg.

Related to the block:

- The risk of vascular injection is high with an interscalene or a stellate ganglion block.
- There is a risk of high absorption — scalp, bronchial mucosa, pleura.
- Single vs. continuous infusion.
- Conduct — frequent aspiration, incremental, test dose, ultrasound use.

Patient factors:

- Renal, liver or cardiac disease — reduced clearance.
- Elderly patients — low clearance.
- Children — low alpha-1 acid glycoprotein (AAG), increases elimination half-life.
- Pregnant — low AAG levels, increased perfusion and absorption.

d) List a few steps that you could take to prevent LAST. 2 marks

- Pre-procedure — risk/benefit, communication, monitoring, labelling syringes.
- During the procedure — frequent aspiration, slower injection, communication with the patient, ultrasound use, Luer connectors.

- Post-procedure — catheters labelled correctly, documentation, ongoing monitoring.

e) How would you manage LAST once it has occurred? 4 marks

AAGBI guidelines, 2010:

- Early diagnosis and suspicion.
- Immediate management:
  - stop injecting;
  - resuscitation — 100% oxygen, CPR;
  - control seizures.
- Treatment:
  - IV lipid emulsion (ILE);
  - continue CPR.
- Follow-up:
  - intensive care monitoring;
  - patient care for future.

f) What are the mechanisms of action of intravenous lipids in LAST? 2 marks

- Lipid sink hypothesis — lipid expands intravascularly and draws down local anaesthetic.
- Enhanced fatty acid metabolism — bupivacaine inhibits fatty acid oxidation, affecting the heart; IV lipids provide fatty acids.
- Others — fatty acids inhibit local anaesthetic binding to cardiac sodium channels; there is a cytoprotective effect by activating protein kinase B; an inotropic effect by increasing intracellular calcium; altered kinetics and shunting to sequestering organs; a cardiotonic effect by positive inotropy and lusitropy (relaxation of cardiac muscle).

References

1. Christie LE, Picard J, Weinberg GL. Local anaesthetic systemic toxicity. *Br J Anaesth Education* 2015; 15(3): 136-42.

Chapter 19

Other topics in general medicine

ANSWERS

Q1 — Mental Capacity Act

a) What are the principles underlying the Mental Capacity Act (MCA) 2005? 5 marks

- Unless proved otherwise, a person must be assumed to have capacity.
- All the practicable help should be offered to a person before you treat them as lacking capacity.
- Just because a person makes an unwise decision, they should not be treated as if they lack capacity.
- If an intervention/decision is made on behalf of a patient who lacks capacity, then it needs to be in their best interest.
- If healthcare professionals have to make a decision for a person who lacks capacity, then the decision must cause the least restrictions of their rights and freedom of action in order to achieve this purpose.

b) How would you define "capacity" with regards to the above act? 2 marks

Capacity is the ability to understand the given information and to use it to make a decision and subsequently communicate the decision made. This has to be done without coercion.

c) How would you assess capacity? 4 marks

The patient must be able to:

- Understand information about the decision.
- Remember that information.
- Use that information to make a decision.
- Communicate their decision by talking, using sign language or by any other means.

d) What has changed in the consent process since the Montgomery's case? 4 marks

- The duty of the medical professional towards the patient about the disclosure of risk was changed after the Montgomery's case.
- The standard for assessing medical negligence has changed from "what the ordinary responsible physician may feel appropriate to inform" to "what a reasonable patient would like to know" after the Montgomery's case.
- Any material risk must now be clearly communicated to the patient during the consent process by the treating physician.

e) Who is responsible for consent? 3 marks

- The individual who performs the procedure is responsible for obtaining a valid informed consent.
- Alternatively, this process can also be delegated to a suitably qualified individual who has adequate knowledge of the procedure being performed and can inform the benefits and risks involved (in accordance with the General Medical Council [GMC] guidelines), so that the patient is able to make an informed decision.
- This information provided should be tailored in terms of its relevance to that particular patient.

f) If you treat a patient without consent, what could be the consequences? 1 mark

- Treating a patient without consent could lead to a conviction for battery (assault).

g) Which medical body has laid down the guidance on the consenting process in the UK and cite this guidance? 1 mark

The General Medical Council: "Consent: patients and doctors making decisions together".

References

1. Orr T, Baruah R. Consent in anaesthesia, critical care and pain medicine. *Br J Anaesth Education* 2018; 18(5): 135-9.
2. Consent to treatment. NHS, 2019. https://www.nhs.uk/conditions/consent-to-treatment/. Accessed on 25th June 2019.

Q2 — Accidental awareness

a) What is accidental awareness under general anaesthesia (AAGA)? 1 mark

Awareness is said to have occurred when the patient has an explicit recall of the intraoperative events associated with or without pain.

b) What is the overall incidence of awareness under general anaesthesia and the estimated awareness incidence for a caesarean section under general anaesthesia as per the NAP5 study? 2 mark

- The overall incidence of patients reporting an incidence of awareness under general anaesthesia is around 1:19,000.
- The estimated awareness incidence in a caesarean section under general anaesthesia is around 1:670 patients.

c) List the monitoring devices that can be used to help reduce the incidence of awareness under general anaesthesia. 2 mark

- Bispectral Index and M-Entropy™ — both provide a processed EEG as a measure of cortical suppression. They give a number (dimensionless index) to be interpreted.
- Narcotrend®.
- aepEX® device — uses auditory evoked potentials to derive the depth of anaesthesia.
- Another technique is the isolated forearm technique.

d) What are the factors contributing to the increased incidence of awareness? 10 mar

- Females > males — 65% vs. 35%, respectively.
- Obese category patients > other (underweight, normal, overweight and morbidly obese groups of patients) categories.

- Surgical specialty — obstetrics (highest incidence), cardiothoracic surgery (second highest).
- Phases of anaesthesia — induction phase (more common) > maintenance phase > emergence phase.
- Induction agents — more common with thiopentone, etomidate, ketamine and midazolam compared with propofol.
- More common with TIVA.
- Reported more with the use of neuromuscular blockers than without them.
- Use of neuromuscular blockers, not monitoring their effects and no reversal of neuromuscular blockers — all increase the risk of awareness.
- It is more likely to happen in patients with a history of awareness under general anaesthesia in the past.
- Other over-representations for awareness in the NAP5 study included early middle-age adults, out-of-hours operating under general anaesthesia and junior anaesthetists managing the case.
- Drug errors including failure of anaesthetic delivery, e.g. malfunction of the TIVA pump.
- Inadequate administration of volatile anaesthetic agent.

e) How would you minimise the chances of awareness in anaesthesia? 5 marks

- Identify risk factors during the pre-assessment stage itself.
- Vigilance during anaesthesia — keep a watch on the physiological parameters (HR, BP, RR, obvious movements, lacrimation).
- Minimise drug errors during anaesthesia.
- Supplementary doses of induction agent in cases of unexpected delay in intubation, e.g. in a difficult intubation.
- Use of neuromuscular monitoring if neuromuscular blockers are used.
- Depth of anaesthesia monitoring if using a TIVA technique.
- Extra caution in certain surgeries prone to awareness, e.g. caesarean section under general anaesthesia, cardiothoracic surgeries, etc.

References

1. Goddard N, Smith D. Unintended awareness and monitoring of depth of anaesthesia. *Br J Anaesth Education* 2013; 13(6): 213-7.
2. Pandit JJ, Cook TM. Accidental awareness during general anaesthesia in the United Kingdom and Ireland. NAP5 summary of main findings and incidences. National Audit Project 5, 2014. https://www.nationalauditprojects.org.uk/NAP5report. Accessed on 25th June 2019.

Q3 — NAP6 report on anaphylaxis

a) List the four common triggers for perioperative anaphylaxis according to the report of the National Audit Project 6 (NAP6) from the Royal College of Anaesthetists. 4 marks

- Antibiotics — 44%.
- Muscle relaxants — 33%.
- Chlorhexidine — 9%.
- Patent blue dye (used in breast surgeries) — 5%.

b) What is the estimated incidence of perioperative anaphylaxis? 1 mark

One in 10,000.

c) Outline the pathophysiological process of anaphylaxis. 5 marks

- Immunologically-mediated response.
- The suspected antigen combines with immunoglobulins (IgE) causing mast cell degranulation with the release of vasoactive mediators (e.g. histamine, tryptase, leukotrienes, prostaglandins, etc.) with its effects on various systems.
- Cardiovascular system — intravascular volume redistribution causing reduced blood pressure associated with reduced cardiac output and reduced coronary perfusion.
- Capillary leak — causing angioedema, laryngeal oedema, urticaria and hypotension.
- Smooth muscle contraction in the respiratory system and abdomen leading to bronchospasm and abdominal pain/cramps, respectively.

d) Describe your management of intraoperative anaphylaxis in an adult patient. 8 marks

- Recognition of anaphylaxis from other differential diagnoses.
- Remove the trigger for anaphylaxis.
- Call for help.
- ABCDE approach, monitoring of oxygen saturation, ECG and non-invasive blood pressure as the minimum requirement.
- Treat life-threatening problems first, e.g. if blood pressure is <50mmHg or cardiac arrest — CPR in accordance with the ALS® algorithm, immediate adrenaline and IV crystalloid boluses.
- The drug of choice is adrenaline — dose 500μg IM (1:1000) or 50μg boluses IV (1:10000) (boluses as needed).
- Consider an adrenaline infusion if needed — administer in monitored settings.
- For refractory hypotension — consider a vasopressin 2 IU bolus and repeat as necessary.
- IV crystalloid fluid boluses — 20ml/kg bolus as needed.
- Second-line drugs — chlorphenamine 10mg IM or a slow IV in adults; hydrocortisone — 200mg IV in adults.
- Serum mast cell tryptase levels — as soon as possible after emergency treatment, 1-2 hours later and 24 hours later (as a baseline).
- Other steps in management:
  - 100% oxygen;
  - if there are circulation problems — flatten the operating table with the legs up;
  - if there are airway and breathing problems — early tracheal intubation in airway obstruction; head up (propped up position) to facilitate ventilation;
  - if the patient has stridor — use an adrenaline nebuliser (400μg/kg);
  - watch for the biphasic response of anaphylaxis;

- observation for 12-24 hours — consider transfer to the ITU if needed;
- appropriate documentation in the notes.

e) What should be done after successful treatment of anaphylaxis? 2 marks

- Referral to an allergy specialist.
- Communication with the patient and family regarding the events and actions taken must be done by the anaesthetists as well as allergy doctors.
- Anaphylaxis education for patients — avoidance of the allergen.

References

1. Mills ATD, Sice PJA, Ford SM. Anaesthesia-related anaphylaxis: investigation and follow-up. *Br J Anaesth CEACCP* 2014; 14(2): 57-62.
2. NAP6 report. Anaesthesia, surgery and life-threatening allergic reactions. National Audit Project 6, 2018. https://www.niaa.org.uk/NAP6Report. Accessed on 25th June 2019.

Q4 — Emergency laparotomy and NELA

An 82-year-old male is listed on the emergency operating theatre list for an urgent laparotomy. He presented with an acute abdomen and pain.

a) What is the 30-day mortality for a patient having an emergency laparotomy? 1 mark

15%.

b) What are the common indications for an emergency laparotomy as per the National Emergency Laparotomy Audit (NELA) 2015? 2 marks

- Intestinal obstruction.
- Perforation.
- Peritonitis.
- Ischaemia.
- Abdominal abscess.
- Sepsis.
- Haemorrhage.
- Colitis.
- Anastomotic leak.
- Intestinal fistula.

c) How would you prepare this patient for anaesthesia? 2 marks

- Risk stratification — history, examination, tests.
- Consider and treat sepsis.
- Antibiotics within the first hour of the diagnosis of sepsis.
- Fluid resuscitation.

d) How would you anaesthetise this patient for an emergency laparotomy? 2 marks

- Secure the airway rapidly, minimising the risks of pulmonary aspiration.
- Haemodynamic stability during RSI and throughout the perioperative period.
- Optimal volume and type of fluids.
- Protective lung ventilation strategies.
- Analgesia.

e) List the postoperative considerations in this patient. 2 marks

- Analgesia — multimodal, regional techniques (central neuraxial, TAP or rectus sheath).
- Intensive care — if predicted mortality is more than 10%.
- Risks of aspiration during extubation.
- Avoidance of hyperglycaemia and optimising nutritional status.

f) As per the third National Emergency Laparotomy Audit (NELA) 2017, what are the nine key standards of care? 6 marks

- CT scan reported before surgery.
- Risk of death documented before surgery.
- Arrival in the operating theatre within a timescale appropriate to urgency.
- Preoperative review by a consultant surgeon and anaesthetist — if the NELA risk of death is >5% (counted as two separate key standards).
- Both the consultant surgeon and anaesthetist should be present in the operating theatre if the risk is >5% (counted as two separate key standards).
- Intensive care admission if the risk of death is >10%.
- Assessment by a geriatrician for a patient >70 years of age.

g) What are the constituents of the Emergency Laparotomy Pathway Quality Improvement Care (ELPQuiC) bundle? 5 marks

- Early assessment and resuscitation.
- Early antibiotics.
- Prompt diagnosis and early surgery.
- Goal-directed fluid therapy.
- Postoperative intensive care.

References

1. Ilyas C, Jones J, Fortey S. Management of the patient presenting for emergency laparotomy. *Br J Anaesth Education* 2019; 19(4): 113-8.

Q5 — Aspiration of gastric contents

A 60-year-old man is having an elective knee arthroscopy and has just aspirated a significant amount of gastric fluid during anaesthesia. He has a supraglottic airway device in place and is breathing spontaneously. His inspired oxygen fraction is 1.0 and the pulse oximeter shows an oxygen saturation of 91%.

a) Describe your immediate management of this patient. 4 marks

- Call for help.
- Rapid sequence induction with cricoid pressure.
- Secure the airway with an ETT.
- Suction the trachea through the ETT before commencing positive pressure ventilation.
- Postoperative ITU care as prolonged periods of mechanical ventilation may be required.
- Early bronchoscopy.
- Early chest X-ray.
- Antibiotics only if pneumonia develops.

b) List the respiratory complications he could develop in the next 48 hours. 2 marks

- Chemical pneumonitis.
- Bacterial pneumonia causing consolidation.
- ARDS.
- Aspiration of solid particulate causes distal atelectasis and large particles cause proximal airway obstruction and hypoxia.

c) What are the possible preoperative risk factors for regurgitation and aspiration of gastric contents in this case? 4 mar

Patient factors:

- Full stomach — inadequate fasting, gastrointestinal obstruction, emergency surgery.
- Delayed gastric emptying — trauma, opioids, pregnancy and labour, autonomic dysfunction as in DM and CRF, raised intracranial pressure, previous GI surgery.
- Incompetent lower oesophageal sphincter — hiatus hernia, reflux disease, morbid obesity, previous upper GI surgery.

Surgical factors:

- Laparoscopy.
- Lithotomy.
- Upper GI surgery.

Anaesthetic factors:

- Light anaesthesia.
- Difficult airway.

Device factors:

- First-generation supraglottic airways with positive pressure ventilation.
- Long duration of surgery.

d) What are the normal physiological mechanisms preventing reflux? 2 marks

Lower oesophageal sphincter (LOS) reinforced by:

- Crura of the diaphragm.
- Acute angle between the stomach and oesophagus.
- Barrier pressure — pressure in the LOS is higher than the gastric pressure.

Upper oesophageal sphincter formed by:

- Cricopharyngeus and thyropharyngeus.

Protective airway reflexes:

- Coughing.
- Laryngospasm.

e) Describe the strategies available to reduce the risk and impact of aspiration of gastric contents in any patient. 5 marks

- Reducing gastric volume:
  - preoperative fasting;
  - nasogastric aspiration;
  - prokinetic premedication.
- Avoidance of general anaesthetic:
  - regional anaesthesia.
- Reducing pH of gastric contents:
  - antacids;
  - H2 histamine antagonists;
  - proton pump inhibitors.

- Airway protection:
  - tracheal intubation;
  - second-generation supraglottic airway devices;
  - prevent regurgitation;
  - cricoid pressure;
  - rapid sequence induction.
- Extubation:
  - awake after the return of airway reflexes;
  - position (lateral, head down or upright).

f) List the summary of recommendations from NAP4 on aspiration. 3 marks

- Assess for aspiration risk before surgery.
- Airway management strategies should be consistent with identified risk.
- The equipment and skills to detect and manage aspiration should be available at all times.
- Rapid sequence induction remains the standard technique for airway protection.
- Those applying cricoid pressure should be trained and practice applying cricoid pressure regularly.
- In cases where tracheal intubation is not indicated, but when a small increase in aspiration exists, second-generation supraglottic airways should be considered.
- Strategies should be used to reduce aspiration at emergence.
- Anaesthetists should be aware of the prevention, detection and management of blood clot aspiration.
- Active measures should be taken when a flat capnography trace occurs when blood has been near the airway.

References

1. Robinson M, Davidson A. Aspiration under anaesthesia: risk assessment and decision-making. *Br J Anaesth CEACCP* 2014; 14(4): 171-5.
2. NAP4. Major complications of airway management in the UK. National Audit Project 4, 2011. https://www.rcoa.ac.uk/nap4. Accessed on 25th June 2019.

Q6 — Phaeochromocytoma

A 45-year-old patient is reviewed in the preoperative assessment clinic prior to surgery to excise a phaeochromocytoma.

a) What are the characteristic clinical features of a phaeochromocytoma? 6 marks

- Pheochromocytomas are catecholamine-secreting tumours of the adrenal medulla.
- Half of them are diagnosed on abdominal scans as an incidental finding.
- Symptoms:
  - classic triad — headache, palpitations and sweating;
  - abdominal pain;
  - anxiety;
  - tremors;
  - lethargy;
  - nausea;
  - visual disturbances.
- Signs:
  - pallor;
  - hypertension;
  - weight loss;
  - hyperglycaemia.

b) Which specific biochemical investigations might confirm the diagnosis of a phaeochromocytoma? 2 marks

Measurement of metanephrine and normetanephrine levels in plasma (more sensitivity) or urine (more specificity).

c) Which specific radiological investigations might confirm the diagnosis of a phaeochromocytoma? 2 marks

- All radiological investigations need to be correlated with the clinical picture.
- MRI abdomen — more commonly used.
- CT abdomen.
- MIBG scan.
- PET scan.

d) How would you pharmacologically optimise the cardiovascular system prior to surgery? 6 marks

- Arterial blood pressure control:
  - preoperative alpha-blockade with doxazosin or phenoxybenzamine, to be started at least 1-2 weeks preoperatively (prior to this if cardiomyopathy or refractory hypertension exists);
  - calcium channel blockade — as an add-on drug if alpha-blockers are not sufficient, e.g. nicardipine 30mg BD.
- Heart rate control/arrhythmia control — use of beta-blockers, e.g. atenolol, metoprolol. Beta-blockade must be started only when complete alpha-blockade is established.
- Circulating volume optimisation — measure the haematocrit to guide this. The gradual control of arterial pressure will allow circulating volume to return to normal over a period of time.
- Myocardial optimisation — optimising tachyarrhythmias and myocardial ischaemia as needed.

e) How would you assess the adequacy of cardiovascular optimisation preoperatively? 1 mark

Arterial pressure readings must be <130/80mmHg consistently before the surgery.

f) Mention the steps in the management of intraoperative hypotension following tumour devascularisation. 3 mark

- Stop hypotensive medications.
- Optimise intravascular fluid volume.
- Noradrenaline infusion if needed — to titrate with blood pressure.
- Vasopressin bolus 0.4 U to 20 U followed by an infusion for refractory hypotension.

References

1. Connor D, Boumphrey S. Perioperative care of phaeochromocytoma. *Br J Anaesth Education* 2016; 16(5): 153-8.

Q7 — TIVA and TCI

a) What are the indications for total intravenous anaesthesia (TIVA)? 5 marks

- A history of severe postoperative nausea and vomiting.
- Risk of malignant hyperthermia.
- Transfer of anaesthetised patients between different environments.
- Patient's choice.
- Anaesthesia outside the operating theatre.
- If using a neuromuscular blocker, this is a disadvantage for the anaesthetised patient or surgeon.
- For airway surgeries with no endotracheal tube, e.g. rigid bronchoscopy with biopsy.
- Neurosurgery — for a smoother induction and awakening.

b) What are the main components of a target-controlled infusion (TCI) system? 3 marks

- Interface for the user — to register the patient's details and the target concentrations.
- Software validated for the given drug to control the infusion.
- Communication between this software and pump hardware.

c) What are the potential patient problems with TIVA? 2 marks

- Awareness risk.
- TIVA methods are not validated in the morbidly obese population; there is a risk of inadequate dosage (TIVA pumps are limited to a BMI of 42 in males and 35 in females).
- Propofol-related infusion syndrome.
- Analgesia and hyperalgesia.
- Accidental overdose in the elderly and frail patients with recommended dosages.

d) How might each of these problems in question c be minimised? 6 marks

- Awareness risk — monitor the depth of anaesthesia, minimise technical errors in the infusion system (e.g. watch for connection issues with IV cannulas), understand the TIVA pharmacology.
- Morbid obesity — the use of ideal body weight in TCI pumps with a supplemental bolus of propofol ready to administer. Use continuous clinical assessment and depth of anaesthesia monitoring to assess the need to administer this additional bolus.
- Propofol-related infusion syndrome — this is rare. Be vigilant for an unexplained metabolic acidosis so that the infusion can be stopped and the anaesthetic maintenance changed to an inhalational method.
- Analgesia and hyperalgesia — use a non-opioid-based analgesic plan for the postoperative period; use local and regional analgesia.
- Accidental overdose in the elderly and frail patients — use slow incremental doses to reach the intended effect site concentration titrated to the haemodynamic and depth of anaesthesia monitor response.

e) What are the potential technical problems with TIVA? 4 marks

- IV cannula malfunction, tubing disconnection, leakage issues — cause a failure of delivery of TIVA.
- A risk of overdose with TIVA drugs in the absence of an antisiphon valve and minimal dead space distal to the TIVA tubing attachment.
- Failure of pump programming with the combined loss of AC and battery power.
- Drug errors with a remifentanil infusion.
- Forgetting to disconnect and flush the TIVA tubing at the end of the case may cause the accidental administration of remifentanil in the postoperative period if the cannula is flushed.

References

1. Al-Rifai Z, Mulvey D. Principles of total intravenous anaesthesia: practical aspects of using total intravenous anaesthesia. *Br J Anaesth Education* 2016; 16(8): 276-80.

Q8 — Obstructive sleep apnoea and STOP-BANG

A patient with obstructive sleep apnoea (OSA) but no other cardiovascular or respiratory comorbidity is scheduled to have peripheral surgery with at least one night stay in the hospital.

a) List all the elements of the STOP-BANG assessment for a patient with suspected OSA. 4 marks

- Snoring — do you snore loudly?
- Tired — do you feel tired, fatigued or sleepy during the day?
- Observed — has anyone observed you stopping breathing during your sleep?
- Blood pressure — do you have high blood pressure or are you on treatment for it?
- BMI — is your Body Mass Index >35kg/m^2?
- Age — are you over 50 years old?
- Neck circumference — is your neck circumference greater than 40cm (16 inches)?
- Gender — are you male?

Scores are marked as yes or no.

b) How is the STOP-BANG assessment used to quantify risk? 3 marks

- A score of 3 or more 'yes' answers — indicates a high risk of OSA although a high proportion of false-positives will be included.
- A score of 5-8 'yes' answers — identifies patients with a high probability of moderate or severe OSA, the group most likely to benefit from particular attention.

c) What are the cardiovascular consequences of OSA? 3 marks

- Arrhythmias, especially atrial fibrillation.
- Increased incidence of atherosclerotic coronary disease.
- Increased incidence of coronary events.
- Development of congestive heart failure.

d) What steps can be taken to minimise perioperative risk in this patient having peripheral surgery? 10 marks

Preoperative assessment and preparation:

- Review of this patient in a dedicated high-risk anaesthetic clinic, rather than on the morning of surgery.
- Ensure an adequate routine preoperative anaesthetic assessment with a special focus on airway assessment.
- Encourage the patient to use CPAP regularly and to bring it into the hospital.
- Explain the reasons for a postoperative overnight hospital admission.

Intraoperative care:

- The use of a local or regional technique may be possible as it is a peripheral surgery.
- If using central neuraxial block, supplement with a long-acting local anaesthetic in the peripheral nerve blocks to ensure longer-lasting postoperative analgesia.
- General anaesthesia may be used if a local/regional block is inadequate for surgery.
- Anticipate a difficult airway and make the appropriate preparations, including considering the use of Optiflow THRIVE™.
- Extubate once fully awake.

Postoperative care:

- CPAP may be required to support the airway with or without supplementary oxygen administration.
- Analgesic regimes used should cause no respiratory depression.
- Local/regional analgesia is preferred for the postoperative period.
- A prolonged period of monitoring may be required especially when the patient is sleeping.
- Care should be provided in an appropriately staffed area that can recognise and manage problems related to OSA.

References

1. Hall A. Sleep physiology and the perioperative care of patients with sleep disorders. *Br J Anaesth Education* 2015; 15(4): 167-72.

Q9 — Postoperative nausea and vomiting

a) List the patient-related risk factors for postoperative nausea and vomiting (PONV). 7 marks

- Female gender.
- Non-smoking status.
- History of motion sickness, PONV or both.
- Low ASA physical status (ASA I-II).
- Preoperative anxiety.
- History of migraine.
- Age — in adults with increasing age, the risk of PONV decreases but in the paediatric population, the incidence of PONV increases with age.

b) What are the anaesthetic-related risk factors for PONV in adult patients? 3 marks

- Use of volatile anaesthetics.
- Use of nitrous oxide.
- Intraoperative and/or postoperative opioid usage.
- Duration of anaesthesia.

c) What are the unwanted effects of PONV in adults? 6 marks

- Delayed patient discharge.
- Increased unanticipated hospital admissions.
- Patient dissatisfaction.
- Suture dehiscence.
- Aspiration of gastric contents.
- Oesophageal rupture.

d) Which non-pharmacological interventions have been shown to be effective in reducing PONV in adults? 2 marks

- Acustimulation of P6 — acupressure/acupuncture/electroacupuncture.
- Hypnosis.
- Aromatherapy.

e) Briefly explain the proposed mechanisms of action of 5-HT3 antagonists such as ondansetron when used as an antiemetic. 2 marks

- Ondansteron is a potent, highly selective, competitive antagonist at 5-HT3 receptors.
- It lacks a dopamine receptor antagonist property.
- The mechanism of action is not clearly elucidated.
- It inhibits 5-HT3 receptors in CNS regions (area postrema, nucleus tractus solitarius, amygdala and dorsal raphe nucleus).
- Ondansetron inhibits 5-HT3 receptors in the peripheral nervous system also; it blocks the depolarisation of vagal afferent nerves and myenteric neurones. This attenuates the 5-HT3 receptor-mediated nociceptive response.

References

1. Pierre S, Whelan R. Nausea and vomiting after surgery. *Br J Anaesth CEACCP* 2013; 13(1): 28-32.

Q10 — Extubation problems

a) List the airway risk factors that may indicate a difficult extubation. 3 marks

- Known difficult airway.
- Restricted access to the airway.
- Airway deterioration secondary to haematoma, oedema, trauma, bleeding, etc.
- Obstructive sleep apnoea/obesity.
- Risk of aspiration.

b) List the patient factors that you can optimise prior to extubation. 4 marks

- Cardiovascular stability needs to be ensured.
- Respiratory factors — gas exchange and establishing a regular breathing pattern.
- Metabolic factors — correct any metabolic/electrolyte abnormalities, e.g. severe hypokalaemia, hypoglycaemia, etc.
- Temperature — correct hypothermia/hyperthermia.
- Neuromuscular block reversal.

c) What other factors can you optimise prior to extubation? 4 marks

- Equipment — airway adjuncts and bite blocks, suctioning of airway.
- Location — it is safer to extubate in the operating theatre environment if needed.
- Skilled assistance — to facilitate a sitting-up position.
- Facilitate monitoring and close observation.

d) Enumerate the strategies that you would employ to manage a high-risk extubation. 5 marks

- Plan — assess and optimise the airway and general risk factors.
- Optimise patient-related and other logistical factors that could contribute to a difficult extubation.
- Perform an awake extubation if the above factors are optimised followed by appropriate monitoring of the patient — by using humidified O_2, high-flow humidified nasal oxygen, epinephrine nebulisation as needed.
- The use of advanced extubation techniques:
  - laryngeal mask exchange technique — replace the tracheal tube with a laryngeal mask to suppress cough and ensure smoother emergence with non-traumatic extubation;
  - use a remifentanil infusion technique — to suppress peri-extubation coughing and to facilitate extubation whilst being awake. A low-dose remifentanil infusion is maintained until extubation;
  - use an airway exchange catheter — the catheter must always be above the carina and not >25cm inside in a typical adult patient.
- The decision to postpone extubation and monitor in an appropriate setting until some of the high-risk factors are stabilised.
- The decision not to perform extubation and go for a tracheostomy instead — for long-term protection of the airway.

e) Outline the steps you would take to exchange an endotracheal tube for a supraglottic airway device (SAD) to aid extubation. 4 marks

- 100% oxygen supplementation to pre-oxygenate.
- Suction through the endotracheal tube.
- Aspirate stomach contents to minimise aspiration risk.
- Use a deeper plane of anaesthetic to aid extubation with minimal coughing.
- Insertion of a supraglottic airway after extubation.

- Connect to the breathing circuit and check for ventilation.
- Check the correct seating of the LMA at the laryngeal inlet with a fibreoptic scope to facilitate the reintubation with an Aintree catheter if needed.

References

1. DAS Extubation guidelines. Difficult Airway Society, 2011. https://das.uk.com/content/das-extubation-guidelines. Accessed on 25th June 2019.
2. Batuwitage B, Charters P. Postoperative management of the difficult airway. *Br J Anaesth Education* 2017; 17(7): 235-41.

Q11 — LASER and laryngeal surgery

A 77-year-old man is scheduled for laser surgery on a laryngeal tumour.

a) What does the term "LASER" stand for? 1 mark

Light amplification by stimulated emission of radiation.

b) What is the character of the light that forms a LASER? 1 mark

An intense beam of monochromatic, non-divergent light.

c) What different types of laser can be used for surgery? 3 marks

- Solid-state laser — Nd-YAG laser — neodymium yttrium aluminium oxide garnet laser.
- Semiconductor laser — GaAs (gallium arsenide) laser.
- Gas laser — CO_2 laser, helium-neon laser, argon laser.

d) How can the risk of an airway fire be minimised? 5 marks

- Ventilating with air or using as minimum oxygen as possible to maintain adequate oxygenation — air-oxygen mixture with <25% O_2 ideally.
- Minimise reflection of the laser beam from surgical instruments — use non-reflective matt-black surfaces.
- Protect other surrounding tissues with wet swabs.
- Instilling normal saline in the cuff of the endotracheal tube.
- Using special purpose laser-resistant endotracheal tubes, e.g. Laser-Flex™ tubes.

e) What measures would you take to protect the staff when a laser is in use? 4 marks

- Label the operating theatre to inform that a LASER is in use.
- Doors should be locked and windows need to be covered in theatres.
- Appropriate eye protection goggles for all staff.
- An appropriate non-water-based fire extinguisher should be made available in the operating theatre.
- Make sure that all the staff members are aware of LASER safety principles and management protocols.
- A laser protection supervisor for every clinical area where it is used.

f) What anaesthetic techniques can be used to allow a tubeless field for laryngeal surgery? 5 marks

- Jet ventilation/high-pressure source ventilation — a rigid bronchoscope with a jet ventilator attachment by various approaches that include:
  - a supraglottic approach;
  - a transglottic approach;
  - a transtracheal approach.
- Maintainence of spontaneous ventilation in general anaesthesia — low-flow oxygen can be delivered distally via a catheter.
- An apnoeic oxygenation technique with general anaesthesia — with high-flow oxygen.
- High-flow nasal oxygen delivery — with warmed and humidified oxygen.
- Use of a smaller endotracheal tube/microlaryngoscopy tube with intermittent positive pressure ventilation.
- Topical anaesthesia along with short-acting strong opioids are useful in these techniques to reduce the degree of response to surgical stimulation.
- TIVA needs to be used in most cases since an inhalational anaesthetic delivery is difficult to control using the above techniques.

g) Give one example of LASER-resistant endotracheal tubes used in airway surgeries. 1 mark

- Mallinckrodt™ Laser-Flex™ tube — double cuff.
- Bivona® foam cuff tube.

References

1. Pearson KL, McGuire BE. Anaesthesia for laryngo-tracheal surgery, including tubeless field techniques. *Br J Anaesth Education* 2017; 17(7): 242-8.
2. Kitching AJ, Edge CJ. Lasers and surgery. *Br J Anaesth CEPD Reviews* 2003; 3(5): 143-6.

Q12 — Cerebral palsy

An 8-year-old child is scheduled for an elective right femoral osteotomy due to impending dislocation of the hip. She has severe cerebral palsy.

a) What is cerebral palsy? 3 marks

Cerebral palsy (CP) is a collective term to describe a group of neurological disorders with varying degrees of motor, sensory and intellectual impairment due to injury to the developing brain.

b) List the causes of cerebral palsy. 3 marks

CP is a pathological injury to the developing foetal or infant brain and this can be congenital or acquired.

Congenital CP (80%):

Foetal pathogenic factors:

- Vascular maldevelopments.
- Congenital genetic/metabolic disorders.
- Foetal trauma.
- Neonatal asphyxia in the peripartum period (6%).
- Low birth weight, prematurity.
- Multiple births, prenatal 'TORCH' infections (toxoplasmosis, rubella, *Cytomegalovirus*, and *Herpes*).

Maternal pathogenic factors:

- Breech presentation.
- Pre-eclampsia.
- Peripartum haemorrhage.
- Maternal hyperthyroidism.
- Foetal alcohol syndrome.

Acquired CP (20%) — develops during the first 2 years of life:

- Intracerebral haemorrhage.
- Viral encephalitis.
- Bacterial meningitis.
- Hyperbilirubinaemia (kernicterus).
- Head injury, neonatal seizures.

c) List the typical clinical features of severe cerebral palsy, with its associated anaesthetic implications. Do this for the central nervous system, respiratory system, musculoskeletal system and gastrointestinal system. 8 marks

Central nervous system:

- Impaired mobility — an inability to assess the cardiorespiratory reserve.
- Impaired intellect, cognition, vision, hearing and speech causing:
  - communication problems; elicit a history from the carers and notes;
  - heightened anxiety and the need for premedication.
- Poorly controlled epilepsy:
  - antiepileptic drug therapy to continue perioperatively;
  - caution with regard to drug interactions.

Respiratory system:

- Chronic lung disease:
  - reactive airway problems;
  - physiotherapy;
  - bronchodilators;
  - antibiotics perioperatively.
- Weak cough, respiratory muscle hypotonia — increased risk of aspiration.
- Scoliosis — restrictive lung defects.

- All these problems can cause pulmonary hypertension, cor pulmonale.

Gastrointestinal system:

- Poor chewing, swallowing, due to pseudobulbar palsies, oromotor dysfunction — lead to malnutrition, dehydration, anaemia and electrolyte imbalances.
- Poor swallowing, failure to clear secretions and GORD — risk of aspiration.
- Constipation and use of laxatives — dehydration and electrolyte imbalance.
- Poor dentition, TMJ dislocation, muscle spasticity — difficult airway.

Musculoskeletal system:

- Fixed flexion deformities, joint dislocations, scoliosis and decubitus skin ulcers:
  - difficult patient positioning;
  - difficult vascular access;
  - difficult to establish invasive monitoring.
- Osteopenic bones — risk of fractures.
- Poorly contracting muscles on incision — increased risk of bleeding.
- Thin skin, very little subcutaneous fat and atrophic muscles — poor temperature regulation.

d) What are the expected problems in providing adequate postoperative analgesia in this patient? 2 marks

- Communication difficulties make the assessment of pain difficult.
- Opioids can cause oversedation, depress the cough reflex and cause respiratory depression.
- Regional techniques are difficult due to scoliosis, contractures and a difficulty in positioning.

- Painful muscle spasms are triggered by hypothermia, anxiety and postoperative pain.
- Muscle spasms are relieved by baclofen, diazepam or midazolam which in themselves cause muscle weakness and respiratory depression.

e) Outline a management plan to optimise analgesia in this patient. 4 marks

- Continuous analgesic regimens are better than intermediate regimens.
- Multimodal analgesia to reduce opioid use.
- Regular paracetamol and NSAIDs.
- Caudal/epidural analgesia — continuous infusion of local anaesthetics and adjuvants like clonidine.
- Femoral/sciatic nerve blocks — continuous infusion of LA through femoral nerve catheters.
- Continue antispasmodic medication.
- Avoid hypothermia and anxiety which precipitate muscle spasms.
- IV opioids and extradural opioids can precipitate respiratory depression; hence, use with caution.

References

1. Prosser DP, Sharma N. Cerebral palsy and anaesthesia. *Br J Anaesth CEACCP* 2010; 10(3): 72-6.

Q13 — Acute pancreatitis

a) List two common causes of acute pancreatitis in the United Kingdom. 1 mark

- Alcohol.
- Gallstones.

b) What are the components of the revised Atlanta criteria 2012 for the diagnosis of pancreatitis? 3 marks

A minimum two of the three criteria need to be satisfied:

- Abdominal pain suggestive of pancreatitis.
- Serum amylase and/or lipase levels >/= three times the upper limit of the normal value.
- Imaging findings consistent with acute pancreatitis — contrast-enhanced CT, MRI or an ultrasound scan.

c) Classify acute pancreatitis according to the severity. 3 marks

According to the updated Pancreatitis Severity Scale (in the Revised Atlanta classification):

- Mild acute pancreatitis — no local or systemic complications.
- Moderately severe acute pancreatitis — the presence of local complications, e.g. a peripancreatic collection or the presence of systemic complications, e.g. exacerbation of chronic pancreatitis or organ failure which is transient (<48 hours).
- Severe acute pancreatitis — persistent single or multiple organ failure for more than 48 hours.

d) What is the role of antibiotics in acute pancreatitis? 2 marks

- Antibiotics are not routinely recommended for prophylaxis or in mild acute pancreatitis.
- Antibiotics should only be considered in infected pancreatic necrosis (suspected or confirmed), systemic sepsis or organ failure.

e) What are the specific principles of managing severe acute pancreatitis in a critical care environment? 7 marks

- ABC approach with supportive management as appropriate.
- Organ support as needed, e.g. ventilatory failure — invasive ventilation and circulatory support with vasopressors as needed.
- Initial fluid resuscitation followed by optimising fluid management.
- Monitoring — arterial blood pressure, ABG, cardiac output monitoring as needed.
- Prevention/early recognition of complications, e.g. optimise fluid management, glycaemic control and avoid nephrotoxic drugs — to minimise acute kidney injury.
- Nutrition — early (within 72 hours) enteral feeding — cheaper, safer, better overall outcome. Parenteral nutrition is considered only if enteral nutrition has failed for 5-7 days.
- Prevent infection.
- Appropriate pain management.
- Treat the cause of pancreatitis where possible.

f) What is the role of surgery and intervention in acute pancreatitis? 4 marks

Surgical management options:

- If there is obstructive jaundice or acute cholangitis — an ERCP +/- sphincterotomy is indicated within 72 hours.

- Mild gallstone pancreatitis — an early cholecystectomy is advised during the same hospitalisation.
- In necrotic pancreatitis — avoid early surgical intervention in the first 2 weeks. A necrosectomy should be delayed for 3-4 weeks to ensure optimal surgical conditions.
- Decompressive laparotomy — if abdominal compartment syndrome develops with respiratory failure.
- Massive haemorrhage due to pseudoaneurysms in pancreatitis — consider radiological management — coil embolisation or balloon tamponade or both.

References

1. Pancreatitis. NICE guideline, NG104. London: National Institute for Health and Care Excellence, 2018. https://www.nice.org.uk/guidance/ng104. Accessed on 25th June 2019.
2. Banks PA, Bollen TL, Dervenis C, *et al*. Classification of acute pancreatitis — 2012: revision of the Atlanta classification and definitions by international consensus. *Gut* 2013; 62: 102-11.
3. Young SP, Thompson JP. Severe acute pancreatitis. *Br J Anaesth CEACCP* 2008; 8(4): 125-8.

Q14 — Postoperative pulmonary complications

a) List the postoperative pulmonary complications that may occur following non-cardiothoracic surgery. 3 marks

- Atelectasis.
- Pneumonia.
- Respiratory failure.
- Pleural effusion.
- Pneumothorax.
- Bronchospasm.
- Aspiration pneumonitis.

b) What are the patient-related (4 marks) and surgery-related (2 marks) risk factors for postoperative pulmonary complications following non-cardiothoracic surgery? 6 marks

Patient-related factors:

Good evidence exists for the following risk factors:

- Age >60 years.
- ASA-PS score of II or more.
- Functional dependency.
- Congestive heart failure.
- Chronic obstructive pulmonary disease.
- Investigation of serum albumin (<30g/L).

Fair evidence exists for the following risk factors:

- Smoking.
- Recent upper respiratory tract infection.
- Obstructive sleep apnoea.
- Alcohol use.

- Weight loss >10%.
- Disseminated cancer.
- Haemoglobin <100g/L.
- SpO_2 <96%.
- Abnormal chest radiograph.

Surgery-related risk factors:

- Prolonged surgery (>3 hours).
- Surgical site — abdominal, thoracic, neurosurgery, vascular, head and neck surgery.
- Emergency surgery.

c) How might anaesthesia contribute to postoperative pulmonary complications? 3 marks

Effect of anaesthetic drugs:

- Hypoventilation.
- Decreased response to hypoxia and hypercapnia.
- Impaired cough.
- Impaired ciliary activity.
- Dry gases cause mucous plugging.

Decrease in FRC:

- Spontaneous ventilation in the supine position — causes basal atelectasis.
- Absorption atelectasis by 100% oxygen.
- Pain after abdominal surgeries causes diaphragmatic splinting.
- Adverse effect on neutrally-mediated diaphragmatic function after abdominal surgeries.

d) What perioperative strategies may you adopt to reduce postoperative pulmonary complications? 5 marks

Preoperative:

- Optimisation of existing cardiorespiratory disease:
  - COPD — continue inhaled beta-2 agonists, anticholinergics or corticosteroids;
  - asthmatics — continue treatment to achieve their best peak flow;
  - OSA — continue CPAP, and weight reduction strategies.
- Early smoking cessation.
- Prehabilitation exercise programmes.
- Perioperative dental care and oral chlorhexidine rinse.

Intraoperative:

- Surgical:
  - minimally invasive surgical techniques;
  - selective use of nasogastric tubes.
- Anaesthetic:
  - lung-protective ventilation strategies;
  - short-acting NMBAs with quantitative monitoring;
  - neuraxial blockade (insufficient evidence);
  - goal-directed fluid therapy (insufficient evidence).

Postoperative:

- Adequate analgesia.
- Early mobilisation.
- Postoperative epidural analgesia.
- Lung expansion techniques.

e) List five lung expansion techniques that could be used postoperatively. 3 marks

- Chest physiotherapy.
- Deep breathing exercises, cough.
- Postural drainage.
- Percussion and vibration, suctioning and ambulation.
- Incentive spirometry.
- Nasal CPAP.
- Nasal high-flow oxygen therapy.

References

1. Davies OJ, Husain T, Sterphens RCM. Postoperative pulmonary complications following non-cardiothoracic surgery. *Br J Anaesth Education* 2017; 17(9): 295-9.

Q15 — Drug approval and levels of evidence

a) What is the process of drug approval and what are the types of studies that must be done for drug approval? 5 marks

- Pre-clinical studies:
  - *in vitro* and animal studies;
  - obtain data on efficacy, toxicity and pharmacokinetics.
- Phase 0:
  - first studies in humans;
  - small numbers of voluntary healthy subjects;
  - microdosing, data on pharmacokinetics and dynamics.
- Phase 1:
  - small group of healthy volunteers;
  - assess dose range — safety, tolerance and maximum dose;
  - data on pharmacokinetics and dynamics.
- Phase 2 :
  - larger groups of patients;
  - case series or RCT trials;
  - assess safety and efficacy.
- Phase 3:
  - RCT and multicentre studies;
  - collect additional data on safety and efficacy;
  - need at least two successful trials for drug approval.
- Phase 4:
  - post-market surveillance.

b) How would you design a study to compare morphine with a newer synthetic opioid in managing pain? 5 marks

- Observation — new drug.
- Review literature — what is already known?
- Generate hypothesis — no difference (null hypothesis).

- Define the aim, objectives and endpoint of the trial — efficacy, safety, adverse effects.
- A prospective study (a prospective study is better than a retrospective study — comparable control, avoids confounding variables).
- Inclusion and exclusion criteria.
- Randomisation.
- Blinding.
- Power calculation from previous studies or pilot study.
- Design consent form.
- Proposed statistical analysis.
- Ethical committee approval — HRA application.
- Study → data → analysis → disperse the findings (publication).

c) How would you evaluate the level of evidence available for a treatment? 5 marks

In the following order:

- Systematic reviews and meta-analysis — level 1.
- RCTs — level 1.
- Cohort studies — level 2.
- Case control studies — level 3.
- Case series — level 4.
- Expert opinion — level 5.

d) How would you stratify the strength of recommendation based on the level of evidence? 5 marks

In the following order:

- Level A — evidence from meta-analyses, systematic reviews and RCTs.
- Level B — cohort and case control studies.
- Level C — case series and case reports.
- Level D — expert opinion.

References

1. Burns PB, Rohrich RJ, Chung KC. The levels of evidence and their role in evidence-based medicine. *Plast Reconstr Surg* 2011; 128(1): 305-10.

Q16 — Oxygenation, lateral decubitus and the alveolar gas equation

a) Name four reasons and explain why anaesthetised patients need more than 21% oxygen. 8 marks

To avoid hypoxaemia due to:

- Abnormal respiratory muscle activity (relaxed airway and spinal muscles, relaxed intercostal muscles, diaphragm displaced cephalad — all three changes lead to an immediate reduction in FRC).
- Formation of atelectasis — a reduced FRC at less than closing capacity in older patients leads to a collapse of the airway. If the FRC is above closing capacity, there are still changes in the chest wall and diaphragm that compress lung tissue. An intrapulmonary pathological shunt results. PEEP is needed to limit this atelectasis.
- Abnormal regional ventilation and perfusion matching in the lungs — IPPV causes more ventilation in ventral regions and increased scattering of V/Q ratios.
- Development of hypercapnia — reduced minute ventilation due to opioids and anaesthetic drugs. Normal reflex ventilator responses are attenuated.

b) A patient is listed for lateral decubitus surgery; how does the V/Q ratio alter in dependent and non-dependent lung regions in different positions with anaesthesia and controlled ventilation? 5 marks

Dependent regions:

- In these areas, V/Q is <1, as there is poor regional ventilation but perfusion is still maintained. Oxygenation is impaired in areas even without atelectasis (V/Q=0 areas). As there are areas of lung with 0> V/Q <1 with the combined shunt through areas of atelectasis, it results in an overall shunt fraction of 10%.

- Increasing FiO_2 by even small amounts (0.3 to 0.4) can correct the adverse effects.

Non-dependent regions:

- Good ventilation but poor perfusion.
- Further induction can lower the cardiac output. Alveolar dead space results which impairs CO_2 removal.
- Hypercapnia results even if minute ventilation is normal.

c) A 48-year-old female is listed for a laparoscopic cholecystectomy. The monitor shows increased $etCO_2$ with signs of hypercapnia. What is the alveolar gas equation and explain how any increase in alveolar PCO_2 will reduce PO_2 in this patient? 7 marks

- $PAO_2 = PiO_2 - (PACO_2/RQ)$.
  where PAO_2 is the alveolar PO_2, PiO_2 is the inspired PO_2, $PACO_2$ is the alveolar PCO_2 (normally the same as $PaCO_2$) and RQ is the respiratory quotient.
- A laparaoscopic procedure with insufflation of gas and reduced ventilation can increase the amount of CO_2 excreted by the lungs. CO_2 will be absorbed from the peritoneum or pleura.
- Using the alveolar gas equation, any increase in alveolar PCO_2 will decrease alveolar PO_2.
- Increasing FiO_2 by a similar amount to increase PCO_2 will prevent this from affecting arterial oxygenation.

References

1. Lumb AB. Why do patients need extra oxygen during a general anaesthetic? *Br J Anaesth Education* 2019; 19(2): 37-9.

Q17 — Effects of smoking

a) What are the clinical effects of cigarette smoking in the following systems? 4 marks

Cardiovascular system:

- 3-4 times increase in coronary heart disease.
- Nicotine — sympathomimetic.
- Carbon monoxide reduces oxyhaemoglobin levels.
- Reduced oxygen supply and increased myocardial demand.
- Arrythmias, lipid profile, plaques, peripheral vascular disease.

Respiratory system:

- The commonest cause of lung cancer.
- Small airway obstruction, reduced FEV1.
- Emphysema.
- Bullous change.
- Bronchoconstriction.
- Increased closing volume.
- Altered V/Q ratio.
- Cough.
- Breath-holding.
- Laryngospasm.
- Impaired mucous clearance.

Gastrointestinal system:

- Relaxes the gastro-oesophageal sphincter.
- Reflux.
- Peptic ulcer.
- Increased metabolism of CYP2E1 (reduced nausea).
- Increased incidence of Crohn's disease (reduced ulcerative colitis).

Other systems:

- Inhibits immune function.
- Poor wound healing.
- Increased wound infection.
- Delayed fracture healing.
- Abnormal bone metabolism.

b) Name four constituents of cigarette smoking that cause damage and their common biological effects in the following. 2 marks

- Polycyclic hydrocarbons — naphthalene, fluorine, phenanthrene — respiratory inflammation, liver dysfunction.
- Nitrosamines — nicotine-derived nitrosamine ketone — procarcinogen, immunosuppressant, interleukin modulation.
- Aza-arenes — quinoline — hepatic carcinogen.
- Aromatic amines — toluidine, anisidine — bladder carcinogen.

c) How would you describe the affinity of carbon monoxide for haemoglobin compared with that of oxygen? 1 mark

- The affinity of CO to Hb is far greater than the affinity of oxygen for Hb.
- P50 for COHb is reduced in comparison with that of the OxyHb dissociation curve.

d) Name any two pharmacological effects of smoking and the effects on various drugs. 2 marks

- Induction of the cytochrome P450 system by nicotine and polycyclic aromatic hydrocarbons (CYP1A1, CYP1A2, CYP2E1).
- Altered metabolism of theophylline, caffeine, haloperidol, propranolol, volatile agents.
- Greater postoperative opioid needs (mechanism not clear).
- Change in nicotinic acetylcholine receptors at the postsynaptic membrane.

e) A 53-year-old male presents to the preoperative assessment clinic for an elective cholecystectomy. Although he presented for cardiac risk and these have been investigated and optimised, the preoperative assessment nurse contacts you as she is worried about the history of smoking 30 cigarettes per day for the last 33 years. As an anaesthetist, what would be your actions in this scenario? 2 marks

- Advice on smoking cessation before surgery, to avoid postoperative complications.
- Even a short period of abstinence helps to avoid some of the adverse effects.
- Combined behavioural support and pharmacotherapy.
- Contact with the local NHS stop smoking service and referral.
- If the patient does not wish to stop smoking, brief advice and support to help them quit.
- VBA tool — very brief advice — three-step approach — ask, advise, act.

f) What are the risks in this patient for anaesthesia considering the association with smoking? 4 marks

Intraoperative complications:

- Increased respiratory adverse events (reintubation after planned extubation).
- Laryngospasm.
- Bronchospasm.
- Aspiration.
- Hypoventilation.
- Hypoxaemia.
- Pulmonary oedema.

Postoperative complications:

- Increased mortality.
- Increased cardiac morbidities.
- Pulmonary and septic complications.
- Increased risk of ICU admission.
- Emergency readmission.
- Longer inpatient postoperative stays.

g) What are the pharmacological options for smoking cessation that are licensed in the United Kingdom? 2 marks

- Nicotine replacement therapy — patches, lozenges, chewing gum, nasal sprays.
- Oral bupropion — nicotinic receptor antagonist with dopaminergic and adrenergic actions.
- Oral varenicline — nicotinic receptor partial agonist.

h) Intraoperatively, this patient develops bronchospasm during his general anaesthesia; what drugs, including dosages, can be used to treat this? 3 marks

- Increase inhaled volatile agent.
- Salbutamol (8-10 puffs into the circuit, 2.5-5mg nebuliser, 250µg slow IV).
- Aminophylline 5mg/kg slow IV.
- Hydrocortisone 100-200mg IV.
- Ketamine 1-3mg/kg/h or 10-20mg bolus.
- Magnesium 1.2-2g IV.
- Adrenaline 10-100µg titrated.

References

1. Carrick MA, Robson JM, Thomas C. Smoking and anaesthesia. *Br J Anaesth Education* 2019; 19(1): 1-6.

Q18 — Oxygenation and hyperoxia

a) What physiological factors determine the rate of fall in arterial oxygen saturation in an apnoeic patient (3 marks), and which patient groups are most likely to show a rapid fall? (4 marks) 7 marks

Factors which determine the rate of fall in oxygen saturation:

- FRC of the patient.
- Preoxygenation.
- Maintenance of a patent airway.
- Metabolic rate.
- Physiological shunt and dead space.
- Haemoglobin concentration.

The patient groups most likely to show a rapid fall are:

- Obese.
- Pregnant.
- Critically ill.
- Neonates and children.

b) How may alveolar oxygenation, prior to intubation, be optimised during a rapid sequence induction (6 marks), and how can its effectiveness be measured? (1 mark) 7 marks

Optimise technique:

- Breathing 100% oxygen at 10-12L/minute using a leak-free mask for 3 minutes using tidal volumes OR 4 vital capacity breaths.

Modify device:

- Use of PEEP with the APL valve.

- CPAP or BiPAP.
- Apnoeic oxygenation:
  - high-flow oxygen through a nasal cannula;
  - THRIVE™.

Optimise position:

- Ramped anti-Trendelenburg position.
- Oxford pillow.

Patient preparation:

- Optimising Hb.
- Optimising respiratory comorbidities — inhalers.
- Maintain a patent airway.

Effective preoxygenation is indicated by an end-tidal oxygen of more than 0.9.

c) What are the possible respiratory complications of prolonged delivery of 100% oxygen? 2 marks

- Absorption atelectasis.
- Abolishes hypoxic pulmonary vasoconstriction.
- V/Q mismatch.
- Acute lung injury.
- Fibrosis.

d) What are the four stages of pulmonary toxicity that occurs due to hyperoxia? 4 marks

There are four stages of pulmonary toxicity. The first three stages constitute ALI and the fourth stage is permanent lung damage:

- Initiation:
  - increased formation of reactive oxygen species;
  - surfactant damage to alveolar epithelial cells and capillary endothelial cell damage.
- Inflammatory stage:
  - destruction of pulmonary lining and migration of inflammatory mediators;
  - hyperpermeability and oedema.
- Proliferative phase:
  - cellular hypertrophy;
  - activation of coagulation cascade — microthrombi;
  - increased secretions from alveolar type II cells.
- Fibrotic phase:
  - collagen deposition;
  - fibrosis.

References

1. Horncastle E, Lumb AB. Hyperoxia in anaesthesia and intensive care. *Br J Anaesth Education* 2019; 19(6): 176-82.
2. Sirian R, Wills J. Physiology of apnoea and the benefits of preoxygenation. *Br J Anaesth CEACCP* 2009; 9(4): 105-8.

Q19 — Antiplatelet medications

a) What are the indications for antiplatelet drugs in clinical practice? 4 marks

The NICE guidelines recommend monotherapy or dual antiplatelet therapy for:

- The primary prevention of atherothrombotic events in people who are at high risk.
- The secondary prevention of atherothrombotic events in people with:
  - acute coronary syndrome (ACS);
  - angina;
  - peripheral arterial disease.
- The secondary prevention of cardiovascular events in people after:
  - myocardial infarction (MI);
  - stent implantation;
  - stroke or transient ischaemic attack.
- The prevention of atherothrombotic events in people undergoing percutaneous coronary intervention (PCI).
- The prevention of pre-eclampsia and its complications.

b) List the agents currently in clinical use. 3 marks

- COX inhibitor — aspirin.
- Phosphodiesterase inhibitor — dipyridamole, cilostazol.
- ADP receptor blocking drug:
  - thienopyridines — ticlopidine, clopidogrel, prasugrel;
  - ADP receptor antagonist — ticagrelor, cangrelor.
- Glycoprotein IIB/IIIA inhibitors — abciximab, eptifibatide, tirofiban.
- PAR-1 blocking drugs — vorapaxar — inhibits thrombin-mediated platelet aggregation.

c) What is the mechanism of action of aspirin and phosphodiesterase inhibitors? 4 marks

Aspirin:

- At low doses (75-300mg) it inhibits the COX-1 enzyme to prevent the formation of thromboxane A2, a platelet aggregator and vasoconstrictor.

Phosphodiesterase inhibitors:

- Prevent the degradation of cAMP.
- Increased cAMP causes the inhibition of platelet activation by increasing the level of calcium ions.
- Inhibit adenosine uptake by platelets.
- Increase the levels of cGMP by PDE5 inhibition and cause vasodilatation.

d) What is the mechanism of action of ADP receptor blocking drugs and GP IIb/IIIa inhibitors? 4 marks

ADP receptor blocking drugs:

- Thienopyridines — bind to ADP receptors and inhibit platelet aggregation.
- ADP receptor antagonists — inhibit ADP-induced signalling.

Glycoprotein IIb/IIIa inhibitors:

- Bind to the GP IIb/IIIa receptors and inhibit platelet aggregation by preventing the binding of vWF and fibrinogen.

e) How may active bleeding be managed following the administration of one of these agents? 5 marks

- A restrictive transfusion management strategy, with transfusion thresholds of haemoglobin <80g/L.
- No antagonists for antiplatelet agents are available.
- The management of significant haemorrhage — tranexamic acid, fibrinogen, factor XIII, desmopressin, platelets and activated factor VIIa.

References

1. Antiplatelet treatment. NICE Clinical Knowledge Summaries. London: National Institute for Health and Care Excellence, 2018. https://cks.nice.org.uk/antiplatelet-treatment. Accessed on 25th June 2019.
2. Ramalingam G, Jones N, Besser M. Platelets for anaesthetists — part 2: Pharmacology. *Br J Anaesth Education* 2016; 16(4): 140-5.
3. Koenig-Oberhuber V, Filipovic M. New antiplatelet drugs and new oral anticoagulants. *Br J Anaesth* 2016; 117(S2): ii74-ii84.

Q20 — Fundoplication and laparoscopic effects

A 35-year-old patient is scheduled for an elective Nissen fundoplication.

a) List and briefly state the reasons for the cardiovascular effects of laparoscopy in the head-up position for a Nissen fundoplication. 7 marks

Cardiovascular effects of positioning:

- Reduced venous return.
- Hypotension.
- Myocardial ischaemia.

Cardiovascular effects of a pneumoperitoneum:

- Increased intra-abdominal pressure.
- Increased systemic vascular resistance from mechanical compression of the abdominal aorta.
- Increased systemic vascular resistance from the production of neurohumoral factors such as vasopressin and activation of the renin-angiotensin-aldosterone axis.
- Compression of the vena cava reduces preload, thus, reducing cardiac output. This can lead to a decrease in arterial pressure, more marked in hypovolaemic patients.

b) What are the respiratory effects of this surgery in the same patient? 4 marks

- Raised intra-abdominal pressure limits diaphragmatic excursion.
- Raised intrathoracic pressure.
- Reduced pulmonary compliance.
- Reduced FRC.
- Pulmonary atelectasis.

- Altered V/Q ratio.
- Hypoxaemia.
- Absorption of insufflated CO_2 leads to an increase in PCO_2.

c) What ventilation strategies can be used to minimise these side effects? 4 marks

- Conventional volume-controlled ventilation increases the risk of barotrauma and high inflation pressures.
- Pressure-controlled ventilation:
  - allows higher instantaneous flow peaks;
  - minimises peak pressures;
  - improves alveolar recruitment and oxygenation.
- The use of titrated levels of PEEP minimises alveolar derecruitment.

d) List any four benefits of laparoscopic surgery. 2 marks

- Reduced incidence of wound infection.
- Quicker recovery times.
- Decreased morbidity.
- Less pain.

e) List the risks of laparoscopic surgery. 3 marks

- Visceral damage.
- Damage to vessels.
- Complications from extreme positioning.
- Acute kidney injury.
- Myocardial ischaemia.
- Cerebral ischaemia.
- Pulmonary atelectasis.
- Venous gas embolism.

References

1. Hayden P, Cowman S. Anaesthesia for laparoscopic surgery. *Br J Anaesth CEACCP* 2011; 11(5): 177-80.

Q21 — Splenectomy

A 26-year-old patient with stage 4B Hodgkin's disease (spread to lymph nodes and other organs) requires an open splenectomy.

a) List the specific factors that are of importance in the preoperative planning for this patient. 6 marks

- Multidisciplinary team management regarding the Hodgkin's disease and its progression — involving the haematologist/oncologist/surgeon/anaesthetist/intensivist.
- Routine preoperative assessment with a focus on systemic involvement from the Hodgkin's disease.
- Assess systemic involvement from the advanced Hodgkin's disease and investigate accordingly — routine bloods, ECG, CXR, CT lungs, pulmonary function tests, echocardiography.
- Assess the patient for systemic complications of chemotherapeutic drugs for the treatment of Hodgkin's disease especially bleomycin.
- If the patient has received radiotherapy, assess for side effects.
- The patient may need irradiated or HLA-matched blood/blood products.
- A vaccination schedule should be planned preoperatively.

b) List the salient features of intraoperative management for this patient. 5 marks

- General anaesthesia with a cuffed endotracheal tube.
- Insert a large orogastric tube to deflate the stomach and aid surgical access.
- Use large-bore intravenous access, as blood loss can be significant.
- Use invasive blood pressure and cardiac output monitoring to guide fluid management.
- Consider pressure control ventilation to avoid barotrauma.

- Anticipate atelectasis and hypoxia due to pulmonary fibrosis from chemotherapeutic agents, and manage with PEEP.
- Avoid high oxygen concentrations to prevent further bleomycin-induced pulmonary damage.
- Antibiotic prophylaxis.
- Venous thromboprophylaxis.

c) Outline the options for providing postoperative analgesia for this patient and give a possible disadvantage of each. 4 marks

- Epidural analgesia — there is a risk of epidural haematoma from preoperative/intraoperative and postoperative haematological issues (thrombocytopenia).
- Morphine PCA/opioids — there is a risk of postoperative respiratory depression and hypoxia if there is ongoing pulmonary fibrosis.
- Non-steroidal anti-inflammatories — renal damage and may increase the risk of bleeding by exacerbating the thrombocytopenia.
- Wound infusion catheters with local anaesthetic — as a solitary mode of postoperative analgesia, this may not be as effective.

d) Which vaccinations should this patient receive and what is the optimal timing of these? 5 marks

Preoperatively (at least 2 weeks before elective surgery) the patient should receive:

- *Haemophilus influenzae* B (Hib) vaccine.
- Meningitis vaccine.
- Pneumococcal vaccine.

Postoperatively, the patient should receive:

- Flu vaccine yearly.
- Pneumococcal vaccine booster every 5 years.

- Travel vaccines.

References

1. Gent L, Blackie P. The spleen. *Br J Anaesth Education* 2017; 17(6): 214-20.

Q22 — Scoliosis surgery

A 15-year-old adolescent girl is listed for surgery for the correction of scoliosis.

a) How would you diagnose adolescent idiopathic scoliosis? 2 marks

- Adam's forward bending test — positive if more than 7°.
- Confirmed on radiographs — Cobb's angle — the degree of the most tilted vertebrae on X-ray of more than 10°.

b) What is the incidence of scoliosis? 2 marks

- Scoliosis affects 1-3% of adolescents.
- Scoliosis with a Cobb's angle greater than 30° affects 0.15-0.30% of adolescents.

c) What are the problems that would result due to scoliosis? 3 marks

- Cosmetic deformity.
- Psychosocial distress.
- Physical problems — back pain, affects cardiorespiratory function.
- Shift of vertebrae.

d) What surgical procedures are available for scoliosis? 2 marks

- Harrington rod instrumentation (increased back pain).
- Posterior spinal instrumentation and arthrodesis (posterior spinal fusion) — using intraoperative skull femoral traction.

e) What specific problems related to anaesthesia should be remembered for these surgeries? 2 marks

- Pain management — intraoperatively and postoperatively.

- Antibiotic prophylaxis and the prevention of surgical site infection (incidence 6.7%).
- PONV.
- Temperature management.
- Blood conservation management.
- Prevention of neurological injury.
- Complications of a prone posture — posterior ischaemic optic neuropathy, stroke secondary to arterial occlusion in the neck, injury from inhibition of venous drainage, peripheral neuropathies.

f) What are the intraoperative management strategies that could be considered for scoliosis surgeries? 6 marks

- Analgesia — multimodal analgesia — paracetamol, anti-inflammatories, opioids, gabapentin.
- Patient-controlled epidural analgesia — remifentanil infusions intraoperatively.
- PONV is a major challenge — multiple prophylactic antiemetics are required.
- Fluid balance — avoid fluid load, but avoid hypoperfusion at the same time (goal-directed fluid therapy).
- Blood loss — intraoperative cell salvage if required, tranexamic acid.
- Somatosensory evoked potentials (SSEPs) monitoring and motor evoked potentials (MEPs) monitoring to prevent neurological complications — may need to avoid inhaled anaesthetics. The use of TIVA with propofol and remifentanil infusions is preferred. Avoid nitrous oxide as it affects the potentials.
- Use neuromuscular agents only for induction/intubation and avoid thereafter to facilitate neurophysiological monitoring.
- A BIS monitor or unprocessed EEG can guide the depth of anaesthesia.
- Avoid the complications of a prone posture.

g) List the effects of anaesthetic agents on neurophysiological monitoring that are used during scoliosis surgeries. 3 marks

- All inhaled anaesthetics may interfere with neurophysiological monitoring.
- Nitrous oxide causes a profound depression in amplitude and a longer latency in SSEPs and MEPs.
- Propofol can affect the accuracy of SSEPs and MEPs, but has less effect than volatile agents.
- Ketamine enhances the amplitude of SSEPs and MEPs with spinal stimulation (but less of an effect on subcortical, peripheral and myogenic responses).
- Neuromuscular blockers are to be avoided during neurophysiological monitoring.
- Opioids like remifentanil can affect neurophysiological monitoring but it is not clinically significant.

References

1. Young CD, McLuckie D, Spencer AO. Anaesthetic care for surgical management of adolescent idiopathic scoliosis. *Br J Anaesth Education* 2019; 19(7): 232-7.

Q23 — Perioperative hypothermia

A 54-year-old male underwent a 4-hour laparotomy procedure and experienced a delayed recovery due to hypothermia.

a) What is inadvertent perioperative hypothermia (IPH)? 1 mark

- Core body temperature <36°C.
- A common consequence of anaesthesia.
- Could increase morbidity and potentially mortality.

b) Describe the physiology of thermoregulation. 3 mark

- Core temperature is strictly controlled by many enzyme and transport mechanisms.
- Input — heat and cold sensors — peripheral in the skin and tissues; central in the spinal cord, brain stem and hypothalamus.
- Cold receptors — A delta fibres.
- Warm receptors — C fibres.
- Both receptors communicate via the lateral spinothalamic tract to the preoptic nucleus of the anterior hypothalamus (or via trigeminal nuclei of the head and neck).
- The posterior hypothalamus maintains a temperature set point between 36.7°C and 37.1°C.
- Cold — vasoconstriction occurs via alpha-1 adrenergic receptors and behavioural changes; this is followed by non-shivering thermogenesis via the beta-3 adrenergic receptors (brown adipose tissue), leading to shivering.

c) Describe the effect of anaesthesia on heat balance. 3 mark

- General anaesthesia — challenges the control system and behavioural responses are abolished.
- The inter-threshold range widens from 0.4 to 4°C.

- Homeostasis is compromised.
- Vasoconstriction and shivering thresholds are further reduced in elderly patients.
- The body cannot respond effectively to multiple causes of heat loss during surgery and anaesthesia.
- There is a triphasic pattern:
  - redistribution causes the first rapid decline in temperature — vasodilation is due to the direct effect of anaesthetics and the indirect effects of a lowered vasoconstriction threshold;
  - linear phase 2 — heat loss exceeds the heat produced from metabolism; heat loss is by radiation (40%), convection (30%), evaporation (25%) and conduction (5%);
  - final plateau phase 3 — maximal vasoconstriction, ongoing heat loss balanced by metabolism.

d) What are the risk factors for IPH? 3 marks

- ASA grades II-V (higher the grade, greater the risk).
- Preoperative temperature <36°C.
- Combined GA + RA.
- Risk of cardiovascular complications.
- Major surgeries.
- Low BMI.
- Age — children and the elderly are more at risk.

e) List a few consequences of IPH. 3 marks

- Surgical site infections (SSIs) — decreased blood flow and oxygen flux to the tissues, reduced superoxide radical production.
- Drug metabolism — volatiles — delayed recovery; hepatic metabolism reduced (propofol, opiates); longer action of neuromuscular block.
- Bleeding — impaired platelet function and coagulation cascade.
- Cardiac events — due to increased catecholamines, increased BP and myocardial workload.

- Shivering — increases postoperative pain, monitoring is not reliable, increased CO_2 production.

f) What steps would you take to prevent IPH preoperatively? 2 marks

- Identify patients at risk.
- Measure core temperature.
- Do not transfer to the operating theatre unless a patient's core temperature is >36°C.
- Patients should be encouraged to walk to the operating theatre where possible (increases metabolism).

g) List the measures that you would take in the operating theatre to prevent IPH. 3 marks

- Induction should not be started until the patient's core temperature is >36°C unless this is an emergency.
- Active warming if the anaesthetic time is >30 minutes (forced air warmer recommended).
- Ambient temperature >21°C.
- Warm IV fluids.
- Humidify respiratory gases.
- Monitor temperature at least every 30 minutes.

h) Name two pharmacological agents with doses that could be used if this patient has post-anaesthetic shivering in recovery. 2 marks

- Pethidine 25mg.
- Clonidine 150μg.
- Doxapram 100mg.

References

1. Riley C, Andrzejowski J. Inadvertent perioperative hypothermia. *Br J Anaesth Education* 2018; 18(8): 227-33.
2. Hypothermia: prevention and management in adults having surgery. NICE clinical guideline, CG65. London: National Institute for Health and Care Excellence, 2008; 2016. https://www.nice.org.uk/Guidance/CG65. Accessed on 4th July 2019.

Q24 — Surgical fires

A 72-year-old gentleman is listed for laser debulking of an upper airway tumour; the procedure has a risk of surgical fire.

a) What are the three components of the fire triad required to form a fire? 3 marks

- Fuel source.
- Ignition source.
- Oxidiser.

b) What are the sources of fire in an operating theatre environment? 2 marks

- Fuels — surgical drapes/gowns, laparotomy sponges, dressings, towels, alcohol-based cleaning solutions, tracheal tubes, digestive gases.
- Ignition source — therapeutic laser, monopolar diathermy, light sources, heated probes, faulty electrical wiring, sparks from drills, etc.
- Oxidiser — gaseous oxygen from anaesthetic machine, auxiliary port, cylinder; nitrous oxide is a strong oxidiser.

c) List the algorithm for fire prevention in the operating theatre. 3 marks

- Is the patient at risk of surgical fire?
  - no — > proceed, frequently reassess;
  - yes — > avoid pooling of alcohol-based skin preparation solutions, communication before cautery. Proceed to next step.
- Does the patient require oxygen supplementation?
  - no — > room air sedation;
  - yes — > next step.

- Do you need FiO_2 >0.3?
  - no — > oxygen below 30%;
  - yes — > secure airway with an ETT or supraglottic device.

(Anesthesia Patient Safety Foundation, 2014.)

d) What safety measures would you consider if you are using a cuffed tracheal tube for a laser surgery in the above patient? 2 marks

- Tube specific to wavelength, optical density and power considered to avoid penetration of the tube.
- Cuff inflated with water or saline (and a small amount of dye such as methylene blue).

e) List the types of lasers used and the tracheal tubes that could be used. 2 marks

- Ar^+ laser — Rusch® LaserTubus™.
- Nd:YAG laser — Rusch® LaserTubus™.
- CO_2 laser — Medtronic, Sheridan, Rusch®.
- KTP (potassium titanyl phosphate) laser — Medtronic, Sheridan.

f) What actions would you take in the unfortunate event of a surgical fire in the airway in this patient? 3 marks

- The best action is to prevent a fire.
- The first priority is to stop the burning process.
- Disconnect the oxygen source and remove the endotracheal tube.
- Pour water or saline over the fire before re-establishing ventilation.
- Examine the airway for remnants of tubes, sponges or instruments that might be still there.
- Rigid bronchoscopy soon to examine the distal airways.
- Consider a transfer to a burns specialist centre.
- Assess for toxicity to carbon monoxide or cyanide.

g) List the actions you would take if the fire occurs outside the airway. 3 marks

- Stop the burning process.
- A team member should announce the fire and stop the surgery.
- Briefly attempt to suppress the fire — dowse with water or saline, and place a wet towel.
- If time has elapsed or the fire is larger, drapes should be removed and the relevant steps should be undertaken in the event of an operating room fire.
- Find an appropriate fire extinguisher, turn off oxidised gases and plan for evacuation.
- The local fire alarm should be activated — visual and audible alarms, close the fire doors, and notify the local fire department.

h) How can we improve the culture of fire safety in operating theatres? 2 marks

- Good communication within the team.
- One should speak up and "Stop the Line" without fear.
- Education and mandatory training.
- Mandatory surgical safety checklist for every case and consider a formal fire risk assessment tool, e.g. the Silverstein fire assessment tool — three risk factors — anatomical location, ignition source and open delivery of oxygen.

References

1. Cowles Jr CE, Culp Jr WC. Prevention of and response to surgical fires. *Br J Anaesth Education* 2019: in press; https://doi.org/10.1016/j.bjae.2019.03.007.

Q25 — Sedation

You are asked to sedate a frightened adult patient for the insertion of dental implants.

a) Complete the table with the different levels of sedation from the American Society of Anesthesiologists' (ASA) continuum of sedation (top row) and the clinical features seen at each level (rows below). 8 marks

Table 19.1

	Minimal sedation/ anxiolysis	**Moderate sedation/ analgesia ('conscious sedation')**	**Deep sedation/ analgesia**
Responsiveness	Normal response to verbal stimulation	Purposeful response to verbal or tactile stimulation	Purposeful response following repeated or painful stimulation
Airway	Unaffected	No intervention required	Intervention may be required
Spontaneous ventilation	Unaffected	Adequate	May be inadequate
Cardiovascular function	Unaffected	Usually maintained	Usually maintained

b) Outline the drugs that may be used and their methods of administration, when providing sedation for this patient. 4 mar

Drugs:

- Benzodiazepines (midazolam).
- Opioids (short-acting, e.g. fentanyl/alfentanil).
- Hypnotics (propofol).
- Inhalational agents (nitrous oxide).

Routes:

- Oral.
- Intravenous.
- Inhalational.

c) What are the best practice principles for providing safe sedation in this patient? 8 mar

- Conscious sedation is considered a safe target state.
- Deep sedation requires the same level of care as general anaesthesia.
- Thorough preoperative assessment.
- Valid consent.
- 2-4-6 fasting (maintaining verbal contact could be difficult and there is a high risk of aspiration).
- Titration of drugs to effect.
- Single-agent titration is easier and safer.
- Effective local anaesthesia.
- AAGBI recommended monitoring.
- Discharge only after meeting the set discharge criteria.
- Sedation practitioners should have formal training and assessment of competencies.
- Practitioners use defined methods of sedation for which they have received formal training.

- Regular audit of practice and outcome.
- Every hospital should have a sedation lead.

References

1. Safe sedation practice for healthcare procedures — standards and guidance. Academy of Medical Royal Colleges, 2013. https://www.rcoa.ac.uk/system/files/PUB-SafeSedPrac2013.pdf. Accessed on 25th June 2019.
2. Thompson J, Moppett I, Wiles M. *Smith and Aitkenhead's Textbook of Anaesthesia*, 7th ed. London: Elsevier, 2019.
3. Allman K, Wilson I, O'Donnell A, Eds. *Oxford Handbook of Anaesthesia*, 4th ed. Oxford: Oxford University Press, 2016.

Q26 — MRI scans

You are asked to transfer an intubated intensive care patient for a magnetic resonance imaging (MRI) scan.

a) What is meant by the terms "MR safe" and "MR conditional" in relation to equipment used in the MRI scanner room? 2 marks

- MR safe — equipment poses no additional risk in the MR environment.
- MR conditional — equipment poses no additional risk in the specified MR environment and with specific conditions of use.

b) What precautions should be taken to prevent burns caused by monitoring equipment used in an MRI scanner? 4 marks

- Use fibreoptic pulse oximeters.
- MRI safe ECG electrodes.
- ECG leads placed in a narrow triangle on the chest.
- High impedance, braided, and short ECG leads (avoid loops).
- NIBP machine with non-ferrous connections.

c) Describe other precautions that you should take while this patient is having an MRI scan. 8 marks

- MR safety check of the patient.
- Transfer on an MRI safe non-ferrous trolley.
- Stabilisation of the patient outside the 5 Gauss MRI scanner area.
- Secure the airway (as there is limited access, especially for upper body scans).
- Tape the pilot balloon with a ferromagnetic spring.
- Use an MRI-compatible anaesthetic machine.
- If an MRI-compatible anaesthetic machine is unavailable, then use a long (appropriate) breathing circuit.

- Use MRI safe/conditional infusion pumps.
- If the pumps are incompatible, then use long infusion lines (with infusion pumps outside the MRI room).
- If invasive monitoring is used, the length of pressure line should be minimised to reduce damping.
- MRI conditional or safe monitors.
- Continuous monitoring of the patient (through the control room).
- Consideration of a delayed response if long breathing circuits and infusion lines are used.
- Planning and preparation for rapid retrieval of the patient out of the MRI scanner in an emergency.

d) List any six relative/absolute contraindications to an MRI scan for any patient. 6 marks

- Aneurysmal clips.
- Ocular implants.
- Cardiac pacemakers.
- ICDs.
- Cochlear implants.
- Implanted neurostimulation systems.
- Prosthetic heart valves.
- Orthopaedic implants.

References

1. Reddy U, White MJ, Wilson SR. Anaesthesia for magnetic resonance imaging. *Br J Anaesth CEACCP* 2012; 12(3): 140-4.
2. Miller R, Eriksson L, Fleisher L, *et al. Miller's Anesthesia*, 8th ed. Philadelphia: Elsevier Saunders, 2015.
3. Davis PD, Kenny G. *Basic Physics and Measurement in Anaesthesia*. Oxford: Butterworth-Heinemann, 2003.

Q27 — Pulmonary hypertension

a) Define pulmonary hypertension. 2 marks

Mean pulmonary artery pressure ≥25mmHg at rest or more than 30mmHg with exercise.

b) List four causes of pulmonary hypertension. 2 marks

- Idiopathic.
- Hereditary.
- Congenital.
- Connective tissue disorders.
- HIV.
- Drug- and toxin-induced.
- Portal hypertension.
- Persistent pulmonary hypertension of the newborn.
- Pulmonary veno-occlusive or pulmonary capillary involvement.

c) What are the symptoms and signs in patients with pulmonary hypertension? 3 marks

- Fatigue.
- Dyspnoea.
- Orthopnoea.
- Palpitations.
- Syncope.
- Signs of right heart failure:
  - hepatomegaly;
  - ascites;
  - abdominal distension;
  - peripheral oedema.

d) What are the specific anaesthetic goals when anaesthetising a patient with pulmonary hypertension? 7 marks

- Avoid hypoxia (high inspired oxygen).
- Avoid hypercarbia (moderate hyperventilation).
- Avoid metabolic acidosis (pH >7.4).
- Reduce venous shunt (alveolar recruitment).
- Avoid hyperinflation of alveoli and pulmonary vessel compression (low tidal volume).
- Avoid hypothermia (active warming).
- Avoid volume overload (goal-directed fluid therapy).
- Avoid stress and a sympathetic response (adequate postoperative pain control).

e) List the pharmacological treatments available for this condition. 6 marks

Intravenous:

- Phosphodiesterase-3 inhibitor (milrinone).
- Phosphodiesterase-5 inhibitor (sildenafil).
- Dobutamine.
- Prostacyclin.
- Prostacyclin analogue (iloprost).
- Sodium nitroprusside.
- Nitroglycerine.

Inhalational:

- Nitric oxide.
- Prostacyclin.
- Iloprost.

Oral:

- Phosphodiesterase-5 inhibitor (sildenafil).
- Oral active prostaglandins.

References

1. Elliot CA, Kiely DG. Pulmonary hypertension. *Br J Anaesth CEACCP* 2006; 6(1): 17-22.
2. Miller R, Eriksson L, Fleisher L, *et al*. *Miller's Anesthesia*, 8th ed. Philadelphia: Elsevier Saunders, 2015.

Q28 — Statistics, reviews and meta-analysis

A recent meta-analysis of Mallampati scoring of the airway found that it had a sensitivity of 60% and a specificity of 70%.

a) Briefly define the terms "systematic review" and "meta-analysis". 4 marks

- A systematic review summarises the results of available carefully designed studies according to a predefined protocol.
- A meta-analysis statistically integrates the results of many studies which are too small or inclusive.

b) Explain what is meant by sensitivity and specificity. 4 marks

- Sensitivity — the ability of a test (positive) outcome to correctly identify the actual positive outcome.
- Specificity — the ability of a test (negative) outcome to correctly identify the actual negative outcome.

c) According to this meta-analysis what is the positive predictive value of Mallampati scoring of the airway and how is it calculated? 2 marks

- 67%.
- Percentage of true positive test results out of the total positive results.

d) What is the possible bias with a meta-analysis? 2 marks

- Publication bias.
- Language bias.
- Replication bias.

e) List the key steps in designing a clinical trial. 8 marks

- Observation.
- Literature review.
- Power calculation.
- Define aim and objectives.
- Generate null or alternate hypothesis.
- Methodology:
  - prospective;
  - inclusion and exclusion criteria;
  - randomisation;
  - blinding;
  - standardisation of protocol;
  - outcome measures;
  - patient information and consent.
- Ethical approval.
- Data collection.
- Statistical analysis.
- Dissemination of results.

References

1. Weekes L, Lawson T, Hill M. How to start a quality improvement project. *Br J Anaesth* Education 2018; 18(4): 122-7.
2. Bland M. *An introduction to Medical Statistics*, 4th ed. Oxford: Oxford University Press, 2015.

Q29 — End-stage renal failure

a) List three of the commonest causes of end-stage renal failure (ESRF) in the United Kingdom. 3 marks

- Diabetes.
- Hypertension.
- Glomerulonephritis.

b) What complications of ESRF are of importance to the anaesthetist? 6 marks

- Fluid and electrolyte abnormalities.
- Altered pharmacokinetics of drugs.
- Accelerated atherosclerosis and ischaemic heart disease.
- Pulmonary oedema.
- Peripheral neuropathy.
- Autonomic neuropathy.
- Delayed gastric emptying.
- Anaemia.
- Immunosuppression.

c) What acute physiological disturbances may be seen in a patient who has just had haemodialysis? 3 marks

- Fluid depletion and reduced intravascular volume.
- Electrolyte disturbances — hypokalaemia.
- Residual anticoagulation from dialysis.

d) What are the key practical considerations when providing general anaesthesia for a patient with ESRF on haemodialysis? 8 marks

- Thorough preoperative assessment and optimisation.
- If on haemodialysis, then dialyse 12-24 hours before the elective procedure.

- Antacid prophylaxis and RSI if there is autonomic neuropathy with gastric reflux.
- Caution with suxamethonium (risk of hyperkalaemia).
- Avoid IV cannulation, invasive lines and a blood pressure cuff on the arm with the arteriovenous fistula.
- Protect the arm with the arteriovenous fistula.
- Dosage adjustment of drugs (renal disease causes reduced protein binding of drugs, which can result in an increased free fraction of drugs).
- Careful induction to avoid hypotension.
- Reduce or avoid drugs with predominant renal excretion.
- Prefer non-depolarising muscle relaxants such as atracurium.
- Caution with opioids with active metabolites.
- Caution with potassium-containing fluids.
- Avoid fluid overload.
- Adequate ventilation to avoid the compounding of respiratory acidosis on metabolic acidosis.

References

1. Rang ST, West NL, Howard J, Cousins J. Anaesthesia for chronic renal disease and renal transplantation. *EAU-EBU Update Series* 2006; 4(6): 246-56.
2. Butterworth JF IV, Mackey DC, Wasnick JD. *Morgan and Mikhail's Clinical Anesthesiology*, 6th ed. New York: McGraw Hill, 2018.
3. Hines RL, Marschall KE. *Stoelting's Anesthesia and Co-existing Disease*, 7th ed. Philadelphia: Elsevier, 2017.

Q30 — Malignant hyperthermia

A healthy 39-year-old male is anaesthetised with a general anaesthetic for a laparoscopic cholecystectomy. As soon as the skin incision is made, it is noted that the core temperature is rising quickly. This is associated with a rise in $etCO_2$ and an increase in heart rate.

a) What are the differential diagnoses in this condition? 4 marks

- Malignant hyperthermia.
- Mechanical causes:
  - inadequate FiO_2;
  - inadequate ventilation;
  - problems with the anaesthetic machine or breathing circuit.
- Surgical:
  - laparoscopy with gas insufflation;
  - tourniquet ischaemia;
  - endocrine emergencies.
- Anaesthetic:
  - inadequate analgesia;
  - anaphylaxis;
  - cerebrovascular event.
- Patient-related:
  - anaphylaxis;
  - sepsis;
  - neuromuscular disorders;
  - phaeochromocytoma.
- Others — serotonin syndrome.

b) What is malignant hyperthermia? 1 mark

A progressive, life-threatening hyperthermic reaction occurring during general anaesthesia.

c) Name some triggers for malignant hyperthermia. 2 marks

- Neuromuscular blockers — suxamethonium.
- Volatile agents — halothane, enflurane, isoflurane, desflurane, sevoflurane.

d) What is the pathophysiology of malignant hyperthermia? 3 marks

- Exposure of the trigger causes dysregulation of excitation — contraction coupling (EC) in the skeletal muscle.
- Changes in ryanodine receptor (RyR) isoforms and dihydropyridine receptors (DHPRs).
- Sustained release of calcium into cytosol.
- Increased metabolic demand for ATP causes an increase in CO_2 production and O_2 consumption.
- A rise in CO_2 stimulates the sympathetic system and the heart rate increases.
- Muscle contraction causes acceleration of heat production and muscle rigidity progresses.

e) How would you manage malignant hyperthermia? 8 marks

- Early diagnosis is the key.
- Get more help.
- Stop the volatile agent, use 100% oxygen, hyperventilate, eliminate all triggers.
- Use activated charcoal filters in the circuit (volatile-free machine).
- Intravenous anaesthesia.
- Dantrolene — start at 2.5mg/kg (mixing in 60ml for each vial is time consuming, and so ask for help by assigning one other person the responsibility to prepare this).
- Further doses of 1mg/kg dantrolene.
- A reaction can recur after up to 14 hours of resolution.
- Switch off warming devices.

- Active cooling measures.
- Blood samples, bladder catheter, CVP catheter.
- Treat hyperkalaemia with dextrose insulin or calcium chloride or haemofiltration (especially in rhabdomyolysis).
- Correct acidosis.
- Treat arrhythmias if any.
- Treat acute kidney injury — diuresis, alkalinise the urine.
- Treat coagulopathy.
- Monitor in intensive care unit.

f) How would you confirm the diagnosis of malignant hyperpyrexia? 2 marks

- *In vitro* contracture testing with a muscle biopsy (European MH group guidelines, 2015).
- DNA sequencing technology.

References

1. Gupta PK, Hopkins PM. Diagnosis and management of malignant hyperthermia. *Br J Anaesth Education* 2017; 17(7): 249-54.

Q31 — Rheumatoid arthritis

A 72-year-old patient with longstanding severe rheumatoid arthritis (RhA) presents for a total knee replacement.

a) Which joints may be affected in RhA? Indicate why this is relevant to anaesthesia care. 4 marks

- Atlanto-axial joint:
  - subluxation occurs with neck movements;
  - spinal cord and/or vertebral artery compression leads to quadriparesis or death.
- Cervical spine ankyloses:
  - restricted movement and difficult airway;
  - difficult central venous access.
- Temporomandibular joint:
  - restricted mouth opening and difficult airway.
- Cricoarytenoid joint and other laryngeal cartilages:
  - dyspnoea, stridor, hoarseness;
  - upper airway obstruction postoperatively.
- Costochondral involvement:
  - decreased thoracic compliance.
- Lumbar and thoracic spine:
  - difficult spinal epidural.
- Hip shoulder and knee joints:
  - difficulty in positioning.
- Joints at wrist and phalanges:
  - difficult IV access;
  - difficult to use PCA.

b) What are the effects of RhA on the following systems? 3 marks

Cardiovascular system:

- Pericarditis, myocarditis, endocarditis.
- Valvular hear disease.
- Left ventricular failure.
- Amyloidosis.
- Raynaud's disease.
- Atherosclerosis and IHD.

Respiratory system:

- Reduced chest wall compliance — costochondral involvement.
- Fibrosing alveolitis — restrictive defect.
- Pleural effusions.

Haematological system:

- Anaemia.
- Thrombocytopenia.
- Leukopenia.

c) List the hepatorenal, neurological and ocular manifestations of RhA. 3 marks

Hepatorenal:

- Splenomegaly.
- Hepatomegaly.
- Chronic renal failure.

Neurological:

- Peripheral neuropathy.
- Autonomic neuropathy.

Ocular:

- Keratoconjunctivitis sicca.

d) List the classes of drugs used to treat RhA. 3 marks

- Drugs providing symptomatic relief:
  - corticosteroids;
  - NSAIDs;
  - opioids.
- Conventional disease-modifying antirheumatic drugs:
  - sulphasalazine;
  - methotrexate;
  - azathioprine;
  - cyclosporin;
  - gold;
  - penicillamine.
- Biological DMARDs:
  - etanercept;
  - infliximab;
  - adalimumab;
  - sarilumab.

e) List two systemic side effects of any three medications that you listed above. 3 marks

- Methotrexate — pulmonary toxicity, hepatic cirrhosis.
- Azathioprine — cholestatic hepatitis, bone marrow suppression.
- Cyclosporin — nephrotoxicity, hypertension.

f) Outline the preoperative investigations that are specifically indicated in this patient and the derangements that each may show. 4 marks

- Full blood count — anaemia, thrombocytopenia, leukopenia.
- Urea and electrolytes — chronic renal failure.
- ECG — IHD, valvular heart disease.
- Chest X-ray — fibrosis, rheumatoid nodules.
- Cervical spine imaging (X-ray and MRI) in the case of peripheral neuropathy or neck pain. MRI shows atlanto-axial instability and spinal cord compression.
- Nasendoscopy — cricoarytenoid involvement, rheumatoid nodules.

References

1. Fombon FN, Thompson JP. Anaesthesia for the adult patient with rheumatoid arthritis. *Br J Anaesth CEACCP* 2006; 6(6): 235-9.
2. Rheumatoid arthritis in adults: management. NICE guideline, NG100. London: National Institute for Health and Care Excellence, 2018. https://www.nice.org.uk/guidance/ng100/evidence/july-2018-evidence-reviews-4903172317?tab=evidence. Accessed on 25th June 2019.

Q32 — Point-of-care gastric ultrasound

a) What is the incidence of pulmonary aspiration of gastric contents in elective general anaesthesia? 1 mark

- 1 in 2000-3000 elective GA.
- Mortality is 20% in-hospital.

b) What is the single most commonly used measure to mitigate the risk of pulmonary aspiration? 1 mark

Adequate fasting before anaesthesia.

c) Describe a few rarely used invasive methods to assess gastric contents and emptying. 3 marks

- Assessment of paracetamol absorption.
- Electrical impedance tomography.
- Radiolabelled diet.
- Polyethylene glycol dilution studies.
- Suctioning of gastric contents via gastric tubes.

d) How can point-of-care gastric ultrasound be used in the assessment of risk for pulmonary aspiration? 2 marks

- Detects the presence of solids and liquids.
- Reports a correlation between the gastric cross-sectional area and fasting times.
- Qualification and quantification of gastric contents.

e) Describe the framework used in the performance of point-of-care gastric ultrasound. 4 marks

I-AIM framework (indication, acquisition, interpretation, medical management framework):

- Indication — when food taken is not clear, medical conditions that delay gastric emptying (diabetes, obesity, medications, etc.).
- Acquisition — device, position, image.
- Interpretation — empty, fluid or solid.
- Medical management — clinical correlation, decision-making — anaesthetic technique, timing of surgery.

f) How would you stratify the risk with the findings of a gastric ultrasound? 3 marks

- Empty gastric antrum — a low risk of aspiration.
- Solid food or thick fluid — a higher risk of aspiration.
- Clear fluid — quantify the amount — accepted upper limit is 1.5ml/kg.

g) List a few conditions where gastric ultrasound might be difficult and explain the reasons. 3 marks

- Obesity — a technical challenge, higher antral cross-sectional area, increased depth at which the antrum is found.
- Pregnancy — a technical challenge, a gravid uterus displaces organs cephalad, difficult identification of antrum, tachypnoea and hyperdynamic circulation makes it further difficult.
- Paediatrics — the use of linear high-frequency transducers.

h) What are the advantages of gastric ultrasound? 3 marks

- Simple.
- Painless.
- Non-invasive.
- Bedside and quick.
- Reliable and replicable.
- Influences anaesthetic technique.

References

1. El-Boghdadly K, Wojcikiewicz T, Perlas A. Perioperative point-of-care gastric ultrasound. *Br J Anaesth Education* 2019; 19(7): 219-26.

Chapter 20

Optional topics
ANSWERS

Q1 — Radical nephrectomy

A 59-year-old gentleman is listed for a radical nephrectomy in the urology theatre.

a) How does a radical procedure differ from a simple nephrectomy? 2 marks

A radical nephrectomy involves the resection of the whole of Gerota's fascia, including the perinephric fat, lymphatics and the ipsilateral adrenal gland.

b) This gentleman has a diagnosis of renal cell carcinoma; what are the genetic or environmental risk factors for renal cell carcinoma? 2 marks

- Twice as common in men than women.
- Common in the seventh decade of life.
- Main risk factor — cigarette smoking (one-third of all cases).
- Obesity, hypertension, asbestos exposure, acquired polycystic kidney disease.

c) This patient has a history of high blood pressure, controlled on ramipril and atenolol. How would you assess him preoperatively and what considerations would be taken into account in the preoperative clinic? 4 marks

- Consider the impact of surgery on renal function in the immediate postoperative period.
- Serum creatinine, calculated eGFR and the assessment of differential renal function using computerised isotope renography will influence the surgical approach and perioperative management.
- The assessment of functional capacity and cardiorespiratory disease severity.
- Non-invasive cardiac stress tests, resting transthoracic echocardiogram and static pulmonary function tests.
- Cavo-atrial tumour extension to be assessed.
- Preoperative arterial embolisation of the kidney to reduce blood loss if needed.
- A multispecialty approach with teamwork.
- Transfusion requirements to be assessed and planned.

d) What are the plans that you would make for the intraoperative management of this gentleman coming in for a radical nephrectomy? 6 marks

- Appropriate vascular access, as determined by the surgical approach.
- If IV access is planned, and the patient will be in a lateral position, IV access should be in the ipsilateral limb to the kidney being removed.
- A low threshold for an invasive arterial cannula.
- Non-invasive monitoring of cardiac output and transoesophageal echocardiography.
- Optimise intravascular fluid therapy through stroke volume optimisation.
- Active warming to prevent hypothermia.
- A rigorous approach to venous thromboprophylaxis.

- Bladder catheterisation is routine.
- Broad-spectrum antibiotics in high-risk patients.
- Leucocyte depleting filter in cell salvage (NICE 2008).
- Care with positioning (to avoid pressure sores, nerve damage, venous pooling, corneal abrasion, venous congestion).
- If there is a change in position, new pressure points should be assessed and protected.
- Position-related ventilation-perfusion mismatch, atelectasis.
- Pneumoperitoneum if a laparoscopic approach is planned.
- Regional block with GA — low thoracic epidural analgesia, paravertebral blocks or wound catheters and local infiltration, TAP blocks.
- If there is veno-caval involvement, cross-clamping can reduce cardiac output.

e) What are the complications after a radical nephrectomy? 4 marks

Immediate complications:

- Vascular injury.
- Splenic injury.
- Bowel injury.
- Pneumothorax.

Early complications:

- Acute renal failure.
- Bowel obstruction.
- Peritonitis.
- DVT.
- Pulmonary embolus.

Late complications:

- Chronic renal failure.
- Incisional hernias.
- Wound infection.

f) What are the postoperative concerns in this patient? 2 marks

- High dependency or critical care environment.
- Continuous thoracic epidural analgesia will need care.
- If there is cavo-atrial disease, the patient will need a critical care bed.
- Fluid management.
- Pain management.
- Electrolyte balance and monitoring of blood tests.

References

1. Chapman E, Pichel AC. Anaesthesia for nephrectomy. *Br J Anaesth Education* 2016; 16(3): 98-101.

Q2 — Burns

A 45-year-old man suffered from a flame burn to his body at his work place.

a) Besides the rule of nine method, suggest two other methods for estimating the total body surface area of burn injury. 2 marks

- Lund-Browder chart.
- Patient's palm area.

b) Clinically, how would you differentiate a partial skin thickness burn (second degree) and full skin thickness burn (third degree)? Please give two clinical signs to contrast the difference. 4 marks

- A second-degree burn is painful while a third-degree burn is painless.
- A second-degree burn appears red with blisters while a third-degree burn appears hard, whitish or charred.

c) Name five clinical signs that may raise your suspicion of an airway burn injury. 5 marks

- Stridor.
- Change of voice.
- Shortness of breath.
- Carbon soot in saliva.
- Oedema of oral pharynx.
- Singed nasal hair, eyebrow.
- Severe facial burn.

d) Name four factors that would affect the amount of fluid resuscitation you offer to a severely burned patient. 4 marks

- Total body surface area.
- Body weight.
- Depth of injury.
- Time of injury.
- Urine output.
- Blood pressure.

e) Apart from total body surface area and depth, what other types of injury would you consider managing in a hospital with a burn facility? Please suggest two conditions. 5 marks

- Site — for example, injuries to the face, neck, perineum, etc.
- Chemical burn.
- Circumferential full-thickness burns of limbs and/or the chest
- Electrical burn.
- Medical comorbidity.
- Burn with inhalational injury.
- Injuries in children and the elderly.

References

1. Bishop S, Maguire S. Anaesthesia and intensive care for major burns. *Br J Anaesth CEACCP* 2012; 12(3): 118-22.
2. Norman AT, Judkins KC. Pain in the patient with burns. *Br J Anaesth CEACCP* 2004; 4(2): 57-61.
3. Fenlon S, Nene S. Burns in children. *Br J Anaesth CEACCP* 2007; 7(3): 76-80.

Q3 — Thoracoabdominal aneurysms

A 47-year-old male presents to the accident and emergency department and has a provisional diagnosis of a thoracic aortic dissection. He is haemodynamically unstable.

a) What are the differences between a true aneurysm, pseudoaneurysm and a dissection? 3 marks

- True aneurysm — permanent dilatation of the aorta at least 50% greater than its original size, involving all wall layers.
- Pseudoaneurysm — rupture through the layers of the aorta, held together by blood and surrounding tissues.
- Dissection — disruption of the intimal layer of the aorta, with bleeding within the wall.

b) What are the indications for elective surgery for a thoracoabdominal aortic aneurysm? 3 marks

- Rupture or acute dissection.
- Symptomatic enlargement — pain or compression.
- Aneurysm enlargement >1cm/year or a rapid increase in size.
- Size >6.5cm or >6cm if there is connective tissue disease.

c) How can you classify thoracoabdominal aneurysms? 2 marks

Crawford classification:

- Extent I — from the left subclavian artery to below the diaphragm.
- Extent II — from the left subclavian artery to the aortic bifurcation.
- Extent III — from the lower half of the descending thoracic aorta to the aortic bifurcation.
- Extent IV — confined to the abdominal aorta.

d) How can you classify aortic dissection? 4 marks

DeBakey classification:

- Type I — ascending portion; involves all of the thoracic aorta.
- Type II — ascending aorta only; stops before the innominate artery.
- Type III — descending segment; starts distal to the left subclavian artery.

Stanford classification:

- Type A — ascending aorta; a more virulent course.
- Type B — distal to the left subclavian artery; medically managed.

e) How would you manage the anaesthetic care for this patient? 8 marks

Preoperative:

- Assess functional capacity.
- Evidence of compression of adjacent structures — dyspnoea/stridor.
- Dysphagia.
- Hoarseness.
- Neurological deficit.

Investigations:

- According to urgency; coronary artery disease.
- CT for compression.
- Airway (double-lumen tube may be needed).
- TOE or TTE.
- Need for cross-clamp.
- Surgical approach.
- Surgery involving the aortic arch — full cardiopulmonary bypass with deep hypothermic arrest.

- Monitoring.
- Spinal cord perfusion maintenance and monitoring.
- CSF drainage to maintain spinal cord perfusion pressure.
- Haemostasis.

Postoperative:

- Pain relief.
- Sedation.
- Maintaining spinal cord perfusion in intensive care.
- Complications.
- Monitoring.

References

1. Agarwal S, Kendall J, Quarterman C. Perioperative management of thoracic and thoracoabdominal aneurysms. *Br J Anaesth Education* 2019; 19(4): 119-25.

Q4 — Free flaps in breast surgery

A 35-year-old woman is listed for a mastectomy and free-flap breast reconstruction for breast cancer.

a) What is the difference between a radical mastectomy and breast-conserving treatment? 2 marks

- Breast-conserving treatment — a wide local excision of the tumour with the addition of radiotherapy or chemotherapy; surgery requires histological confirmation of a minimal margin (5mm) of normal tissue excised around the tumour.
- Only 30% need a full mastectomy, the reasons being multifocal disease, inflammatory breast cancer, and prior radiation of the breast, etc.

b) How does sentinel lymph node biopsy differ from axillary lymph node dissection? What are the specific risks of sentinel biopsy? 4 marks

- Sentinel lymph nodes are the first nodes or group of nodes that drain from the primary cancer and are most likely to contain metastatic disease. After injection of radioisotopes, the nodes with highest radioactive signals are removed.
- There are risks with the two dyes that are used (isosulfan blue and patent blue V) — associated with IgE-mediated anaphylactic reactions (overall risk of anaphylaxis is 1% and 0.17% for more serious reactions). NAP6 showed that patent blue V is the fourth most common cause for anaphylaxis perioperatively. Methylene blue is safer but it interferes with pulse oximetry and causes postoperative confusion.

c) What are the different types of flap used for reconstruction after breast tumour excision? 4 marks

- Reconstruction can be immediate or delayed; it can be done using prosthetic or autologous material.
- Prosthetic — a one- or two-staged procedure; tissue expanders are placed under the pectoral muscles and are usually made of silicone.
- Autologous — pedicled (rotational) flaps of tissue (skin, fat and muscle with their accompanying vessels) or free flaps (harvested from the donor site and transferred).
- Pedicle flap — a TRAM (transverse rectus abdominis myocutaneous) flap is the most common; an LD (latissimus dorsi) flap is used if there is a high risk of failure secondary to diabetes or smoking.
- Free flap — a DIEP (deep inferior epigastric perforator) flap spares rectus abdominis and solely uses skin and fat; a microsurgical anastomosis is required and they are often prolonged procedures.

d) What are the causes of flap failure and what physiological goals are important for a healthy free flap outcome? 5 marks

Flap failure:

- Flap failure — 1 in 100 pedicled back flaps fail; 1 in 1000 pedicled TRAM flaps fail.
- The vascular supply is cut off, due to various reasons including hypovolaemia, hypothermia, a pressure effect, oedema, surgical causes, haematoma/bleeding, infection in the wound, tissue breakdown and necrosis, etc.

Goals:

- Avoid hypothermia, hypovolaemia and vasoconstriction.
- Maintain good perfusion of the flap.
- Adequate ventilation of the lungs with a normal PCO_2 and PO_2 will improve perfusion.

- Avoid excess IV fluids to reduce the incidence of tissue oedema after surgery.
- Postoperative flap monitoring — HDU for at least 24 hours and flap monitoring is continued for a number of postoperative days.
- May need a heated room to improve flap perfusion.

e) What are the important anaesthetic considerations for this type of surgery? 5 marks

- Preoperative — a high level of anxiety should be allayed.
- Optimise comorbidities.
- Chemotherapeutic agents can affect the anaesthetic, e.g. cyclophosphamide and doxorubicin can prolong the QT interval and cause cardiotoxicity. Haematopoietic side effects and bleeding risk should be assessed.
- Intravenous access in the contralateral arm to the side of surgery.
- Haemodynamic monitoring as needed.
- Positioning is of prime importance.
- Adequate postoperative analgesia.
- Regional anaesthetic techniques in combination with GA.
- Thoracic paravertebral block, thoracic epidural, pectoral nerve block PECS I and II, serratus anterior plane block, transversus thoracic plane block, local infusion analgesia.

References

1. Sherwin A, Buggy AJ. Anaesthesia for breast surgery. *Br J Anaesth Education* 2018; 18(11): 342-8.

Q5 — Endovascular aneurysm repair

A 79-year-old man with a 6cm infrarenal abdominal aortic aneurysm is to undergo an endovascular aneurysm repair (EVAR). He is known to have chronic obstructive pulmonary disease.

a) What are the advantages of an EVAR compared with an open repair of the aneurysm for this patient? 6 marks

- Improved short-term survival benefit.
- Reduced morbidity.
- Minimises the complications related to laparotomy with a big incision.
- Shorter duration of the procedure, hence a reduced anaesthetic time.
- Options of performing under regional anaesthesia and local anaesthesia are available for some EVARs.
- Less haemodynamic fluctuations.
- Reduced metabolic stress response.
- Less chances of bleeding, blood transfusions and related complications.
- Early ambulation, thereby minimising the complications of immobility.
- Reduced length of hospital stay.

b) Which is the most important modifiable risk factor for the formation, progression and rupture of an abdominal aortic aneurysm (AAA)? 1 mark

Smoking.

c) What are the strongest predictors for rupture of an AAA? 2 marks

- Maximum diameter of the AAA — increased risk >5cm diameter.
- The annual rate of expansion of the aneurysm.

d) List the risk factors for acute kidney injury (AKI) during any EVAR procedure. 5 marks

- Pre-existing problems — chronic renal disease, diabetes mellitus, age >70 years, cardiac failure.
- Reduced renal blood flow during the procedure.
- IV contrast medium-related kidney injury and repeat contrast exposure in the next 7 days.
- Hypotension during the procedure.
- Dehydration in the perioperative period.
- Bleeding.
- Graft displacement can block renal blood flow for that time.
- Complex EVAR, e.g. fenestrated or branched grafts.
- Exposure to nephrotoxic drugs in the perioperative period with ACE inhibitors, aminoglycosides, etc.

e) Enumerate the perioperative measures to prevent AKI following EVAR. 4 marks

- Ensure hydration is good — adequate fluid replacement and maintenance of intravascular volume with urine output monitoring.
- Limit the amount of contrast medium injection.
- Maintain a baseline mean arterial pressure.
- IV N-acetyl cysteine in the perioperative period.
- IV sodium bicarbonate injections.
- Stop all nephrotoxic drugs 24 hours prior to the procedure until the AKI risk subsides.
- Early involvement of the nephrologist in the perioperative period on suspicion of AKI.

f) What percentage of patients develop post-implantation syndrome and what is it comprised of? 2 marks

- 30-40% of patients develop post-implantation syndrome.
- Fever, leucocytosis and a raised CRP — in the absence of sepsis.

References

1. Nataraj V, Mortimer AJ. Endovascular abdominal aortic aneurysm repair. *Br J Anaesth CEACCP* 2004; 4(3): 91-4.
2. Al-Hashimi M, Thompson J. Anaesthesia for elective open abdominal aortic aneurysm repair. *Br J Anaesth CEACCP* 2013; 13(6): 208-12.
3. Kasipandian V, Pichel AC. Complex endovascular aortic aneurysm repair. *Br J Anaesth CEACCP* 2012; 12(6): 312-6.

Q6 — Orthognathic surgeries

A 24-year-old lady is listed for a bimaxillary osteotomy.

a) What are the indications for orthognathic surgery? 2 marks

- Cosmetic.
- Functional improvement.
- Obstructive sleep apnoea.

b) Name any three other types of orthognathic surgeries. 3 marks

- Sagittal split of the mandible.
- Horizontal Le Fort I osteotomy of the maxilla.
- Combined maxillary and mandibular surgery.
- Le Fort II and III surgeries.
- TMJ surgery.

c) What would be your perioperative airway concerns with such a patient? 6 marks

Preoperative airway concerns:

- Plan for difficult airway management due to:
  - congenital syndromes — Treacher Collins syndrome, Apert syndrome;
  - severe malocclusion;
  - TMJ pathology;
  - previous orthognathic surgery.
- Patients may suffer from obstructive sleep apnoea.

Intraoperative airway concerns:

- Problems of a shared airway — tube displacement, tube obstruction, tube damage.

- Nasal intubation is required:
  - look for patency of the nostrils;
  - fix the ETT with minimal distortion of the soft tissues of the face;
  - nasal intubation may be difficult in patients with previous surgeries.
- If nasal intubation proves impossible, the alternatives are:
  - submental intubation;
  - retromolar intubation;
  - tracheostomy.
- Damage to the ETT during an osteotomy:
  - reintubation may be very difficult in this situation;
  - all the adjuncts used to manage the airway at induction should be available to manage this problem;
  - a throat pack can restore ventilation if the damage is limited to the cuff and pilot balloon.
- NPSA guidelines on throat packs should be followed.

Postoperative concerns:

- Ensure the airway is clear of blood and debris.
- Extubate awake.
- Minimise coughing and straining at extubation to prevent bleeding.
- Gentle removal of the nasal tube to prevent displacement of bones.
- Withdraw nasal tube partially so it functions as a nasopharyngeal airway.
- Restricted access to the airway due to intermaxillary fixation.
- Postoperative complications:
  - airway obstruction — haematoma and soft tissue swelling;
  - bleeding from the nose;
  - respiratory depression.

d) How can blood loss be minimised in this case? 3 marks

- Positioning the patient head up.
- Ensuring there is no impediment to venous drainage.

- Induced hypotension.
- Infiltration of epinephrine-containing local anaesthetic solutions.

e) What are the clinical advantages in using remifentanil for this operation? 2 marks

- Good intraoperative analgesia.
- Rapid titration is possible for intermittent high stimulation during surgery.
- Used for induced hypotension to minimise blood loss.
- Accelerated wake up and recovery.
- Smooth emergence.

f) What precautions would you take to reduce the risk of a retained throat pack post-surgery? 4 marks

- Do not insert a throat pack if it is not required.
- If the throat pack is a surgical requirement, the surgeon should verbally communicate with regard to insertion and removal of the throat pack.
- If the throat pack is an anaesthetic requirement, the anaesthetist should verbally communicate with regard to insertion and removal of the throat pack.
- The throat pack should have a radiopaque line and should be a counted surgical sponge.
- One visual check should be implemented:
  - throat pack is attached to the airway device;
  - part of the throat pack is left protruding out of the mouth;
  - a label is attached on the patient or the airway device.
- One documentary check should be implemented. Record the time of insertion and removal on the:
  - white board;
  - surgical count record.

- The anaesthetist should communicate with regard to the removal of the throat pack to the recovery staff.

References

1. Beck JI, Johnston KD. Anaesthesia for cosmetic and functional maxillofacial surgery. *Br J Anaesth CEACCP* 2014; 14(1): 38-42.

Q7 — Perioperative dental damage

a) List any six anaesthetic factors that predispose to perioperative dental damage. 6 marks

- Difficult airway predictors:
  - prominent incisors;
  - Mallampati grade 3 or 4;
  - inter-incisor gap <5cm;
  - limited head and neck movement;
  - limited mandibular subluxation;
  - receding mandible;
  - obesity BMI >35kg/m^2.
- Direct laryngoscopy; tracheal intubation.
- Placement of double-lumen tubes.
- Biting during emergence.
- Forceful removal of tracheal tubes/supraglottic airways.
- Vigorous oropharyngeal suctioning.

b) Name any four dental factors that predispose to perioperative dental damage. 4 marks

- Restorative dental work on any crowns, veneers or prostheses are at risk, especially:
  - anterior restorations;
  - brittle restorative materials, e.g. some ceramics or composite resin;
  - recent restorative/orthodontic treatment.
- Pre-existing dental pathology, previous root canal treatment.
- Periodontitis, caries.
- Isolated teeth.
- Mixed dentition (children aged 5-12).

c) You have anaesthetised a 22-year-old man and you notice a missing front tooth after intubation. What would be your initial management of this situation? 6 marks

- Laryngoscopy and retrieval of the missing tooth using Magill's forceps.
- If the tooth cannot be retrieved:
  - imaging/chest radiograph to determine aspiration into the lungs or oesophagus;
  - if aspirated into the tracheobronchial tree, refer to ENT or a thoracic surgeon.
- If retrieved:,
  - replant into the socket immediately, but do not replant in children, the immunocompromised or those with severe periodontal disease;
  - if it is not possible to reimplant the tooth, place it in a storage medium like cold saline or milk immediately to maintain viability;
  - refer to the dentist/maxillofacial team at the hospital.
- Explanation of the events provided to the patient when fully awake.
- Documentation in the patient's notes.
- Datix reporting.

d) How would you follow this patient up? 4 marks

A Duty of Candour letter which involves:

- An apology to the patient for the dental damage.
- Reassurance that the matter is being investigated.
- Arrange a meeting with the patient to discuss any issues and provide an explanation of the event.

Most of these cases can be settled informally as the cost of defending cases in court is disproportionately high compared with the cost of dental repairs.

References

1. Abeysundara L, Creedon A, Soltanifar D. Dental knowledge for anaesthetists. *Br J Anaesth Education* 2016; 16(11): 362-8.

Q8 — Perioperative medicine and prehabilitation

A 68-year-old male presents to the preoperative assessment clinic for a radical prostatectomy. He is a known hypertensive on ramipril 10mg, bisoprolol 2.5mg and a GTN spray as required. He complains of shortness of breath and, rarely, palpitations on moderate exercise as per his history. He smokes 10 cigarettes per day. His Body Mass Index is 42.3kg/m^2. He has a sedentary lifestyle and drinks five units of alcohol per week. Due to his executive job, his activities are restricted.

a) What is the role of perioperative medicine in this person presenting for a major surgery? 2 marks

- Meets the individual needs of complex patients through all the stages of their surgical journey.
- Provides a multidisciplinary single point of contact team.
- Uses the best available evidence to improve outcomes.
- Shared decision-making is the key.
- An opportunity to make lifestyle modifications as the goal of surgery acts as a catalyst for positive behavioural changes.
- An individualised, procedure-specific model of postoperative care.

b) What is the role of cardiopulmonary exercise testing (CPET) in this individual and what data does it provide? 2 marks

- It is a marker of mitochondrial respiration (coupling of external to internal respiration).
- Individualised assessment of cardiorespiratory function and fitness.
- Four key stages — cardiodynamic, increased cellular respiration, steady state and incremental work phases.
- Nine-panel plot of data representing cardiovascular and ventilatory performance.
- Anaerobic threshold, peak VO_2, ventilatory equivalents ($VE/VECO_2$).

c) What simple bedside tests can you do for this purpose before the CPET in the assessment clinic? 2 marks

- 6-minute walk test.
- Shuttle test.
- Stair climb test.

d) Name any two risk stratification tools used for surgical outcomes. 2 marks

- Portsmouth Physiological and Operative Severity Score for the enUmeration of Mortality and morbidity (P-POSSUM).
- Surgical Outcome Risk Tool (SORT).
- American College of Surgeons National Surgical Quality Improvement Program (ACS NSQIP) risk calculator score.

e) If there is adequate time to prepare in the patient described above, what techniques of prehabilitation can you use? 4 marks

- Preoperative exercise programmes improve outcomes by enhancing the body's ability to withstand the surgical stress response.
- Nutritional optimisation — avoids muscle deconditioning, fatigue, impaired immunity and poor wound healing.
- Psychological interventions to reduce anxiety and stress.
- Lifestyle modification — advice to stop smoking, address the issue of the patient's obesity and alcohol avoidance or reduction.

f) What other comorbidities could be managed in the prehabilitation clinic? 2 marks

- Preoperative anaemia.
- Frailty management.
- Control of blood pressure.
- Diabetes management.

g) What fluid management technique would you use intraoperatively in the operating theatre? 2 marks

- Goal-directed therapy (GDT).
- A radical prostatectomy can cause major blood loss.
- Haemodynamic monitoring.
- Evidence-based algorithms for fluid management.

h) What concerns would you have in the postoperative period for this patient and what techniques would you use for optimal recovery? 4 marks

- Fluid management — monitoring and replacing blood and fluid loss.
- Enhanced recovery after surgery (ERAS) programme — procedure-specific pathways.
- Pre-emptive model of postoperative care planning.
- Pain management — multimodal, opioid-sparing approaches.
- Early physiotherapy and mobilisation.
- The avoidance of postoperative cognitive dysfunction.

References

1. Schonborn JL, Anderson H. Perioperative medicine: a changing model of care. *Br J Anaesth Education* 2019; 19(1): 27-33.

Q9 — Carotid endarterectomy

A 56-year-old man is listed for a carotid endarterectomy 10 days after suffering a cerebrovascular accident.

a) What are the advantages of performing this procedure under regional anaesthesia? 4 marks

- Direct real-time neurological monitoring — the patient acts as the monitor.
- Avoids the associated risks of airway intervention.
- A reduced incidence of the use of shunts.
- A decreased length of hospital stay.
- A reduced risk of postoperative haematoma as it allows arterial closure at normal arterial pressures.

b) What are the disadvantages of using regional anaesthesia for this procedure? 4 marks

- Risks are associated with regional anaesthesia/nerve blocks.
- An increased risk of myocardial ischaemia due to patient stress/anxiety.
- Limited access to the airway during surgery.
- It is only suitable for a cooperative patient who is able to lie flat.
- There is the possible need to convert to GA during surgery.

c) What local or regional anaesthetic techniques may be used? 3 marks

- Local infiltration.
- Superficial and/or deep cervical plexus block.
- Cervical epidural.

d) How can the patient's risk of perioperative cerebrovascular accident be minimised? 6 marks

- Monitoring cerebral blood flow — awake patient/transcranial Doppler/stump pressure/EEG/SSEP/NIRS.
- Deploying a temporary artificial shunt to maintain ipsilateral blood flow.
- Avoiding cardiovascular instability and using invasive arterial blood pressure monitoring.
- Reducing the risk of perioperative thromboembolism by the use of antiplatelet and anticoagulant drugs.

e) Following this procedure, what other specific postoperative complications may occur? 3 marks

- Myocardial ischaemia.
- Heart failure.
- Wound haematoma.
- Cerebral hyperperfusion syndrome — hypertensive encephalopathy.

References

1. Ladak N, Thompson J. General or local anaesthesia for carotid endarterectomy? *Br J Anaesth CEACCP* 2012; 12(2): 92-6.

Q10 — Renal transplant

A patient is scheduled to receive a cadaveric renal transplant.

a) What would be the salient features for preoperative investigation and optimisation of this patient, specific to chronic kidney disease? 8 marks

- History of comorbid illness:
  - diabetes mellitus;
  - hypertension;
  - hypercholesterolaemia;
  - ischaemic heart disease;
  - staging of chronic kidney disease;
  - functional capacity/exercise tolerance.
- Preoperative investigations:
  - full blood count (anaemia/infection);
  - urea and electrolytes;
  - ECG;
  - chest X-ray;
  - detailed cardiac investigations such as echocardiography/CPET/ coronary angiography.
- Medication history:
  - high-dose ACE inhibitors should be withheld perioperatively unless there is left ventricular dysfunction;
  - multiple antihypertensives may be in use such as calcium channel blockers, ACE inhibitors, angiotensin receptor antagonists, alpha-2 agonists;
  - beta-blockers, statins and aspirin should not be stopped perioperatively;
  - continue diuretics in the perioperative period;
  - antiplatelet agents used may impair platelet function and prolong bleeding times.

- Dialysis assessment:
  - blood samples to be taken before and after dialysis to assess volume status, acid base and electrolyte balance;
  - assess the patient's native urine output and volume of fluid removed at each session;
  - dialysis prior to transplantation may cause intraoperative haemodynamic instability but also reduces plasma potassium, corrects acidosis and reduces the need for post-transplantation dialysis.

b) Intraoperatively, how could you optimise the function of the transplanted kidney? 6 marks

- Maintain a mean arterial pressure of 90mmHg (adjusted higher for untreated hypertensives). This preserves residual renal function, reduces delayed graft rejection and the need for post-transplantation dialysis.
- Maintain normotension at the time of graft arterial clamp removal to optimise graft perfusion.
- Maintain a CVP of 12-14cm H_2O at the time of graft perfusion.
- Cardiac output monitoring to guide fluid management.
- Liberal fluid administration at the beginning of surgery but keeping total infusion volumes less than 2.5L.
- Some centres use pharmacological agents such as mannitol and/or dopamine.
- Blood transfusion with a transfusion target of 70g/L will improve oxygen delivery to the transplanted kidney.

c) List three options to manage this patient's postoperative pain. 3 marks

- Renal dose morphine PCA — 0.5mg morphine bolus with a 5-minute lockout.
- Fentanyl PCA.
- Oxycodone.
- Epidural analgesia.

d) List the common postoperative analgesic drugs to be avoided or used with caution. 3 marks

- Non-steroidal anti-inflammatory drugs are contraindicated — they inhibit the synthesis of prostaglandins and thus reduce renal blood flow and glomerular filtration autoregulation.
- Cyclo-oxygenase 2 inhibitors should be avoided.
- Paracetamol should be avoided and used with caution as its sulphur and glucuronide conjugates may accumulate leading to elevated levels of serum creatinine.

References

1. Mayhew D, Ridgway D, Hunter JM. Update on the intraoperative management of adult cadaveric renal transplantation. *Br J Anaesth Education* 2016; 16(2): 53-7.

Q11 — Head and neck cancer and free flap transfer

A 54-year-old patient with a base of tongue cancer presents for a hemiglossectomy and radial forearm free flap reconstruction.

a) List any four aetiological factors implicated in head and neck cancers. 2 marks

- Smoking.
- Alcohol.
- Chewing tobacco.
- Poor oral hygiene.
- Exposure to wood dust.
- Human papilloma virus transmission linked to orogenital sex.

b) Which specific factors must the anaesthetist consider when assessing this patient prior to surgery? 3 marks

- Airway assessment and management strategies.
- Optimisation of comorbidities especially due to smoking and alcohol intake.
- Nutritional assessment and optimisation.
- Perioperative management of alcohol dependence.
- Risk prediction and shared decision-making.

c) What are the preoperative airway considerations? 3 marks

- Often present with a difficult airway.
- Changes to the voice, dysphagia, orthopnoea, and recent onset of snoring may indicate airway obstruction.
- Preoperative radiotherapy makes both face-mask ventilation and laryngoscopy difficult.
- Awake nasal endoscopy gives a real time view of the upper airway and larynx.

- Radiological imaging with CT MRI helps to determine a potential obstruction.
- A nasal ETT may be required.
- Plan postoperative airway management — may require a tracheostomy.

d) What are the causes of impaired nutrition in these patients? 2 marks

- Poor dietary habits (e.g. alcoholism).
- Dysphagia.
- Cancer cachexia.
- Systemic effects of chemotherapy.
- Radiation mucositis.

e) How is the nutritional status optimised in the perioperative period? 1 mark

- Nutritional screening at presentation and specialist dietician input throughout their care.
- Nutritional supplements — oral, NG feeds or a percutaneous gastrostomy.
- Management of refeeding syndrome on reintroduction of feeds.
- Alcohol-dependent patients should be considered for active in-patient withdrawal treatment for at least 48 hours and to optimise electrolytes, haematology and nutrition.

f) What scoring system is recommended to predict cardiac risk in the perioperative period? What is the risk associated with head and neck surgeries? 2 marks

- The Revised (Lee) Cardiac Risk Index is recommended to predict cardiac risk.
- Major head and neck surgeries are intermediate-risk (1-5%) surgeries.

g) List the benefits of a free flap reconstruction. 2 marks

- Better cosmetic appearance.
- Better functional results.
- Protection against infection.
- Flaps can be taken from a distant site.

h) What are the absolute contraindications for a free flap transfer and why? 2 marks

- Sickle cell disease.
- Untreated polycythaemia rubra vera.

These are contraindicated because of the high risk of flap failure due to microcirculatory sludging and thrombosis.

i) What are the intraoperative anaesthetic considerations? 3 marks

- 15-20° head-up tilt to improve venous drainage.
- Access to the head and neck is limited and long ventilator tubing and vascular access lines are required.
- Long-duration surgery and so pressure points must be padded.
- Central venous lines — use femoral vein catheters or peripherally placed central catheters as surgery may involve neck dissection.
- Goal-directed fluid therapy based on cardiac output monitoring to avoid flap oedema.
- Bladder temperature measurement to avoid the use of a probe in the surgical field.
- Remifentanil infusion.
- Dexamethasone to reduce airway oedema and PONV.

(All the factors responsible for the success of free flap surgeries are applicable here and are dealt with in a previous question — Optional topics, Q4.)

References

1. Ahmed-Nusrath A. Anaesthesia for head and neck cancer. *Br J Anaesth Education* 2017; 17(12): 383-9.

Q12 — Direct oral anticoagulants

A 71-year-old male is scheduled for an elective abdominal aneurysm repair. Thoracic epidural analgesia is planned perioperatively. The patient is on rivaroxaban and aspirin.

a) What are the oral anticoagulants that you are aware of? 1 mark

- Warfarin.
- Newer or direct oral anticoagulants (DOACs), e.g. dabigatran, rivaroxaban, apixaban, edoxaban.

b) What are the advantages and disadvantages of warfarin as compared with direct oral anticoagulants (DOACs)? 2 marks

Advantages:

- Wide range of indications.
- Safety — well known.
- Cheap and widely available antidote.
- Preferred in high-risk patients.
- Easily monitored.
- No GI upset.
- Single daily dose.

Disadvantages:

- Need for monitoring.
- Highly variable dosing.
- Increased need for bridging.
- Interactions with food and drugs.
- Slow onset, long half-life.
- Increased risk of intracranial bleed, life-threatening bleed.

c) Name a few indications for DOACs. 2 marks

- VTE prevention after elective hip or knee replacement.
- Secondary prevention or treatment of DVT or PE.
- Stroke and systemic embolism prevention in non-valvular AF.
- Prevention of adverse outcomes after acute management of ACS with raised biomarkers.

d) List the mechanism of action of oral anticoagulants. 2 marks

- Warfarin — inhibits epoxide reductase, which is needed to recycle vitamin K and produce gamma-carboxylated coagulation factors — an indirect mechanism of action.
- Direct oral anticoagulants — quick onset and offset due to a direct mechanism of action:
  - dabigatran — prodrug, directly inhibits thrombin (factor II);
  - rivaroxaban, apixaban — direct inhibitors of factor Xa.

e) How long should you withhold oral anticoagulants perioperatively? 2 marks

- Warfarin — withhold for 5 days (bridging is needed if there are risk factors).
- DOAC — variable duration; if the surgery has a low bleeding risk and there is normal renal function, stop the DOAC 24 hours before surgery. If the surgery has a high bleeding risk, withhold the DOAC for 2-4 days.

f) When would you stop a DOAC before neuraxial anaesthesia? 2 marks

- In very high-risk interventions as the associated bleeding can be devastating.
- Five half-lives are recommended before a neuraxial block (American Society of Regional Anesthesia and Pain Medicine [ASRA] guidelines, 2015).

- Omit rivaroxaban and apixaban for 72 hours (ASRA guidelines, update 2018).
- Check the level of anti-factor Xa or its activity if less than 72 hours.
- If creatinine clearance is >30ml/min, dabigatran should be stopped for 3-5 days; if less than 30ml/min, then do not perform a neuraxial block.
- European guidelines suggest two half-life intervals.

g) When would you consider warfarin bridging and how would you organise this in a patient who takes warfarin? 2 marks

- Warfarin should NOT be stopped if there is a low bleeding risk.
- Patients at low risk of VTE should NOT be bridged.
- Bridging should only be used in cases of high risk of VTE or on an individual case basis with an intermediate risk.
- Bridging — stop the warfarin 5 days before surgery. When the INR is <1.5, start heparin. LMWH is predictable, convenient and efficacious (1.5mg/kg/day).

h) How would you bridge a DOAC? 2 marks

- There is no need for bridging for a DOAC.
- The duration to withhold is short and the effect upon reinitiation is rapid; there is no procoagulant effect.

i) Which group of patients would you consider as high risk for perioperative thrombotic risk? 1 mark

- Mechanical heart valve patients.
- Atrial fibrillation.
- Previous/risk of VTE.

j) What tests would you use to test the efficacy of an anticoagulant? 2 marks

- Warfarin — prothrombin time (PT) or INR.
- Rivaroxaban — anti-factor Xa chromogenic assay.
- Dabigatran — thrombin time (TT), HemoClot® thrombin inhibitor assay.

k) How would you reverse the action of an oral anticoagulant? 2 marks

No/minor bleeding:

- Discontinue anticoagulant.
- Spontaneous resolution.
- Vitamin K for warfarin.

Severe bleeding:

- Discontinue.
- Supportive care.
- Activated charcoal if within 3 hours of ingestion.
- Dialysis for dabigatran.
- Consider a DOAC reversal agent.
- Prothrombin complex concentrate for rivaroxaban and apixaban.
- Vitamin K for warfain.
- Consider recombinant factor VIIa.
- Consider tranexamic acid.

References

1. McIllmoyle K, Tran H. Perioperative management of oral anticoagulation. *Br J Anaesth Education* 2018; 18(9): 259-64.
2. Anticoagulants, including non-vitamin K antagonist oral anticoagulants (NOACs). NICE key therapeutic topic, KTT16. London: National Institute for Health and Care Excellence, 2016, 2018. https://www.nice.org.uk/advice/ktt16. Accessed 8th July 2019.

Q13 — Regional anaesthesia for the eye

a) List the nerves supplying the orbit. 2 marks

Sensory supply (provided by the ophthalmic division of the trigeminal nerve) by three branches:

- Lacrimal.
- Frontal.
- Nasociliary.

Motor supply:

- Oculomotor nerve.
- Trochlear nerve.
- Abducens nerve.

b) What are the contraindications to regional anaesthesia for the eye? 5 marks

Absolute contraindications:

- Patient refusal.
- Local anaesthetic allergy.
- Localised infection at the injection site.

Relative contraindications:

- Poor patient compliance.
- Inability to lie flat/still.
- Positioning difficulties.
- Communication problems.
- Gross coagulopathy.
- Globe perforation/trauma.

c) What is the dose and mechanism of action of hyaluronidase, added to the local anaesthetic mix for eye blocks? 2 marks

- Hyaluronidase causes hydrolysis of hyaluronic acid, a component of the extracellular matrix.
- Advantages — faster onset and a better quality of block.
- Dose — 5-70 IU/ml.

d) Describe the guidance on the use of anticoagulants and antiplatelet medications in patients scheduled for eye surgery. 5 marks

Current joint guidelines are from the Royal College of Anaesthetists and Royal College of Ophthalmologists:

- Continue antiplatelets and anticoagulants in patients scheduled for cataract surgery as day-case patients. Ensure the INR is within the therapeutic range.
- There is no clear evidence to guide in the case of more complicated eye surgery (vitreous surgery, oculoplastic surgery and glaucoma surgery). A multidisciplinary approach should be adopted, and a consensus of opinion sought.
- Postpone elective surgery in patients who have had recent therapeutic cardiac interventions and who are on dual antiplatelet therapy.

e) List any six NICE recommendations (on the day of surgery) to prevent wrong lens implants. 6 marks

Use a checklist, based on the WHO safety checklist, modified to include the following cataract surgery checks, to ensure that:

- The person's identity has been confirmed and matches information in:
  - the consent form;
  - the biometry results;
  - the person's medical notes.

- The eye to be operated on has been checked and clearly marked.
- There is only one intraocular lens in the operating theatre, that matches the person's selected lens type and prescription.
- At least one additional identical intraocular lens is in stock.
- Alternative intraocular lenses are in stock in case the selected lens needs to be changed if there are complications during surgery.
- At least two members of the team, including the surgeon, have previously checked the appropriateness, accuracy and consistency of all:
  - formulas;
  - calculations;
  - intraocular lens constants.

References

1. Cataracts in adults: management. NICE guideline, NG77. London: National Institute for Health and Care Excellence, 2017. https://www.nice.org.uk/guidance/ng77. Accessed on 25th June 2019.
2. Anker R, Kaur N. Regional anaesthesia for ophthalmic surgery. *Br J Anaesth Education* 2017; 17(7): 221-7.

Q14 — Penetrating eye injury and regional block

A healthy 32-year-old male with an ASA I physical status score was involved in a road traffic accident and suffered a penetrating eye injury.

a) What factors determine the intraocular pressure in a healthy eye? 5 marks

- Rate of production of aqueous humor.
- Rate of drainage of aqueous humor.
- Any resistance to the outflow of aqueous humor at the trabecular network.
- Vitreous humor volume.
- Choroidal blood volume.
- Extraocular muscle tone.

b) What key points would you need to know when assessing this patient preoperatively? 3 marks

- General medical history.
- Fasting status.
- Thorough physical examination (in view of trauma).
- Investigations as needed.

c) The patient requires urgent surgery. Discuss your specific intraoperative management. 4 marks

- Avoid factors that could cause a raised intraocular pressure.
- Avoid pressure on the eyeball.
- Inadequate depth of anaesthesia raises intraocular pressure.
- RSI in view of delayed gastric emptying.
- Rocuronium may be preferable over suxamethonium.
- Adequate muscle relaxation before attempting intubation.
- Avoid straining, bucking and coughing on the tube.

- Neutral or slight head-up position.
- Avoid hypoxia and hypercarbia.
- Avoid hypertension.

d) What are the contraindications to perform a regional block in an elective ophthalmic surgery? 5 marks

- Axial length more than 26mm.
- Perforated eye.
- Infected eye.
- Patient refusal.
- Grossly abnormal coagulation.
- Severe reaction or allergy to local anaesthetic drugs.
- Confusion and an inability to communicate.
- Uncontrolled tremor.
- Patient unable to lie flat.

e) What different types of regional block are suitable for ophthalmic surgery? 3 marks

- Retrobulbar anaesthesia.
- Peribulbar anaesthesia.
- Sub-Tenon block.
- Topical anaesthesia.

References

1. Anker R, Kaur N. Regional anaesthesia for ophthalmic surgery. *Br J Anaesth Education* 2017; 17(7): 221-7.
2. Local anaesthesia for ophthalmic surgery: Joint guidelines from the Royal College of Anaesthetists and the Royal College of Ophthalmologists. https://www.rcophth.ac.uk/wp-content/uploads/2014/12/2012-SCI-247-Local-Anaesthesia-in-Ophthalmic-Surgery-2012.pdf. Accessed on 25th June 2019.

3. Nouvellon E, Cuvillon P, Ripart J. Regional anesthesia and eye surgery. *Anesthesiology* 2010; 113(5): 1236-42.
4. Murgatroyd H, Bembridge J. Intraocular pressure. *Br J Anaesth CEACCP* 2008; 8(3): 100-3.

Q15 — Robotic surgeries

a) What are the preoperative considerations for a patient who is listed for robotic surgery? 3 marks

- Thorough preoperative assessment.
- Consideration for the position of the robot in theatre.
- Consideration for the operating table position.
- Account for the whole team's experience with robotic surgery.

b) What are the main physiological considerations in robotic surgery procedures? 3 marks

- Effects due to laparoscopic surgery (pneumoperitoneum, CO_2 absorption).
- Effects due to patient positioning (on haemodynamics, ventilation, intracranial pressure).
- Effects due to prolonged surgery (pressure, hypothermia).

c) What are the main anaesthetic considerations for robotic surgery? 8 marks

- Clear communication with the team.
- Consider anaesthetising on the operating table.
- Accounting for limited space and access to the patient.
- Consider steep positions needed during surgery and plans to restrain.
- Consider haemodynamic and ventilator effects from a pneumoperitoneum and positioning.
- Avoid pressure injury (from a prolonged position; from robotic arms).
- Planning and preparation to take the robotic arms out in an emergency before moving the patient.
- Large-bore venous access.
- Consideration for invasive monitoring.
- Ergonomic consideration of positioning of lines and monitors.

- Adequate depth of anaesthesia.
- Muscle relaxation is paramount.
- Maintain body temperature.
- Apply enhanced recovery principles.
- Multimodal analgesia.

d) What are the possible risks and complications associated with robotic surgery? 4 marks

- Peripheral neuropathies.
- Corneal abrasions.
- Pressure and friction injuries to skin.
- Compartment syndrome with prolonged flexed limb positioning (affecting circulation), especially in lower abdominal and pelvic surgeries.
- Rhabdomyolysis.
- Thromboembolism.
- Oedema (corneal, cerebral, airway).
- PONV from a pneumoperitoneum.

e) List four specialty surgeries that could be done with robotic surgery. 2 marks

- General surgical (fundoplication, bariatric, colorectal).
- Urological (nephrectomy, prostatectomy, cystectomy).
- Gynaecological (radical hysterectomy, salpingo-oophorectomy).
- Cardiothoracic (CABG, VATS).

References

1. Ashrafian H, Clancy O, Grover V, Darzi A. The evolution of robotic surgery: surgical and anaesthetic aspects. *Br J Anaesth* 2017; 119(S1): i72–i84.
2. Joshi GP. Anesthesia for laparoscopic and abdominal robotic surgery in adults. UpToDate. https://www.uptodate.com/contents/anesthesia-for-laparoscopic-and-abdominal-robotic-surgery-in-adults/print. Accessed on 25th June 2019.
3. Lee JR. Anesthetic considerations for robotic surgery. *Korean J Anesthesiol* 2014; 66(1): 3-11.

Afterword

We, the authors, hope that this book has been helpful for your exam preparation. As we said in the beginning, this is not a textbook and it should be used only as an exam preparation guide. Medical science and guidelines keep changing, so please refer to recent appropriate guidelines for clinical practice.

Each candidate has their own exam revision technique and YOU are the person to find this technique and work accordingly. Please make sure you are aware of the vital topics that could come up in CRQ exams and revise appropriately.

For the final FRCA exams, it is important that you read the last 5 years of *BJA Education* topics, NICE guidelines in anaesthesia/critical care/pain, AAGBI guidelines, MHRA recommendations, NPSA patient safety alerts, NAP audit summaries and similar important ones.

Please read the question well; if they ask for any five causes, for example, you are not going to achieve more marks by writing many! Similarly, CRQs test your knowledge and its application: read the question thoroughly and answer specifically to what is being asked.

This book by itself is by no means sufficient as a source of knowledge. However, it certainly will highlight the more important topics and point you in the direction of the references used for these topics. Remember, this is an exam preparation guide that will help you to revise if used appropriately.

Please make sure that you have also read the following important topics:

1. Recent NICE guidelines in anaesthesia including "Routine preoperative tests for elective surgery" (NG45), "Depth of anaesthesia monitors" (DG6), "Sedation in children and young people" (CG112), "Blood transfusion" (NG24), "Venous thromboembolism in over 16s: reducing the risk of hospital-acquired deep vein thrombosis or pulmonary embolism" (NG89).
2. AAGBI guidelines, especially the recent ones such as "Guidelines for day-case surgery", "Perioperative care in people with dementia", "Consent for anaesthesia" (Jan 2017), "Provision of anaesthetic services in magnetic resonance units" and other relevant guidelines.
3. National Audit Projects (NAPs) — especially NAP4, NAP5 and NAP6.
4. RCoA guidelines, e.g. safe sedation guidelines.
5. NELA report, 2018.
6. MBRRACE UK reports, 2018.
7. JBDS-IP guidelines — "Management of adults with diabetes undergoing surgery and elective procedure: improving standards", 2016.
8. The professional duty of candour — GMC guidance.
9. Important clinical trials, e.g. Poise trial, CRASH 2 trial, ENIGMA trial, etc.
10. Cochrane reviews.
11. Emergency tracheostomy management — Resuscitation Council guidelines UK; Difficult Airway Society guidelines.
12. Recent ALS, APLS and ATLS guidelines.

Finally, we wish you all the very best for your examination.

Dr. Pradeep Mukund Ingle